Preface

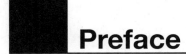

This new edition of the Workbook has been written to solidify a student's awareness of his or her grasp of the topics presented in Surgical Technology Principles and Practice, seventh edition. The questions have been specifically designed to challenge students' strategic thinking skills and to get them to think creatively about scenarios that are commonplace in the modern operating room. The following exercises have been used to meet these goals:

- **Key Terms**. The most important key terms are presented to enhance clarification. Students are asked to differentiate between two terms that are commonly confused and whose precise definitions are key to understanding important concepts.
- **Short Answer** questions apply knowledge learned from the text to a variety of situations.

- **Matching:** These exercises allow students to define and categorize words within a specific area of surgical technology practice. This in turn enhances memorization of each term's meaning and significance.
- **Multiple choice** questions provide a way to differentiate and define information.
- **Labelling** exercises reinforce important anatomy concepts that a surgical technologist should be familiar with.
- **Case Studies** have been carefully written to improve students' critical thinking skills and challenge them to look at clinical situations from various points of view. The case studies also provide a basis for group discussion and knowledge sharing.

Workbook for

Surgical Technology: Principles and Practice

Seventh Edition

Prepared by:

Joanna Kotcher Fuller, BA, BSN, RN, RGN, MPH
Technical Consultant in Surgical, Medical,
and Public Health Response in Conflict Environments
Edinburgh, United Kingdom

ELSEVIER

ELSEVIER

3251 Riverport Lane
St. Louis, Missouri 63043

PRINCIPLES AND PRACTICE
SEVENTH EDITION

ISBN: 978-0-323-39474-1

Notices

Knowledge and best practice in this field are constantly changing. As new research and experience broaden our understanding, changes in research methods, professional practices, or medical treatment may become necessary.

Practitioners and researchers must always rely on their own experience and knowledge in evaluating and using any information, methods, compounds, or experiments described herein. In using such information or methods, they should be mindful of their own safety and the safety of others, including parties for whom they have a professional responsibility.

With respect to any drug or pharmaceutical products identified, readers are advised to check the most current information provided (i) on procedures featured or (ii) by the manufacturer of each product to be administered and to verify the recommended dose or formula, the method and duration of administration, and contraindications. It is the responsibility of practitioners, relying on their own experience and knowledge of their patients, to make diagnoses, to determine dosages and the best treatment for each individual patient, and to take all appropriate safety precautions.

To the fullest extent of the law, neither the Publisher nor the authors, contributors, or editors assume any liability for any injury and/or damage to persons or property as a matter of products liability, negligence or otherwise, or from any use or operation of any methods, products, instructions, or ideas contained in the material herein.

Senior Content Strategist: Nancy O'Brien
Content Development Manager: Ellen Wurm-Cutter
Senior Content Development Specialist: Maria Broeker
Publishing Services Manager: Deepthi Unni
Project Manager: Nadhiya Sekar
Design Direction: Muthukumaran Thangaraj

Printed in the United States of America

Last digit is the print number: 9 8 7 6 5 4 3

Contents

1 The Surgical Technologist

Student's Name _____

KEY TERMS

Provide the definition of each term.

1. Allied health professional: _____

2. AMA: _____

3. AORN: _____

4. AST: _____

5. Certification: _____

6. Continuing education: _____

7. CST: _____

8. CST-CFA: _____

9. Licensure: _____

10. National Certifying Examination for Surgical Technologist: _____

SHORT ANSWERS

Provide a short answer for each question.

11. What are the differences between the titles TS-C and CST?

    _____

    _____

    _____

    _____

12. What are the educational options for students who want to be surgical technologists?

    _____

    _____

13. Why is it important for a practicing surgical technologist to participate in continuing education?

    _____

    _____

14. Name three areas of potential employment for a graduate surgical technologist.

    _____

    _____

1

15. What are the necessary requirements for a surgical technologist to renew his or her certification?

_____

_____

_____

_____

16. Why must a surgical technologist have good organizational skills?

_____

_____

_____

_____

17. What are the educational requirements for a surgical technologist to become a surgical first assistant?

_____

_____

_____

_____

MULTIPLE CHOICE

Choose the best answer to complete the question or statement.

18. The stated goals of a career ladder include all of the following, *except:*
    a. Improve patient care
    b. Promote accountability
    c. Encourage employer recognition of the surgical technologist
    d. Encourage employers to provide a standard salary for surgical technologists

19. The nonsterile member of the surgical team is called the _____.
    a. Technologist
    b. Scrub
    c. Circulator
    d. Surgeon

20. The surgical technologist who works in a hospital or other facility that provides 24-hour care is usually required to:
    a. Take a break every hour
    b. Take emergency call
    c. Work a 24-hour shift
    d. Work overtime

21. The role of the surgical technologist does not include:
    a. Educator and preceptor
    b. Participant in leadership and management
    c. Repair of surgical instruments and medical devices
    d. Specialist in the use and care of surgical instruments

SHORT ANSWER

22. Explain in your own words what *task integration* means.

_____

_____

_____

_____

_____

2 Communication and Teamwork

Student's Name _____

KEY TERMS

Differentiate between the terms.

1. Aggression vs. assertiveness: _____

   _____

   _____

   _____

2. Consensus vs. groupthink: _____

   _____

   _____

   _____

3. Lateral abuse vs. vertical abuse: _____

   _____

   _____

   _____

4. Receiver vs. sender: _____

   _____

   _____

   _____

5. Tone vs. body language: _____

   _____

   _____

   _____

6. Cultural beliefs vs. cultural competence: _____

   _____

   _____

   _____

7. Chain of command vs. social hierarchy: _____

   _____

   _____

   _____

Provide a short answer for each question or statement.

8. What are environmental barriers to communication?

_____

_____

_____

_____

9. Briefly explain three other types of barriers to communication.

_____

_____

_____

_____

10. Briefly explain the phrase "touch is almost never neutral."

_____

_____

_____

_____

11. Why is it important to set boundaries in communicating with patients and their families?

_____

_____

_____

_____

12. What are some of the consequences of a shortage of personnel in the operating room?

_____

_____

_____

_____

13. What are the elements of positive listening skills?

_____

_____

_____

_____

14. What is a team?

_____

_____

_____

_____

15. What is verbal abuse?

_____

_____

_____

_____

16. Withholding information from a work colleague is one form of abuse. Provide an example where withholding information can harm the other person.

_____

_____

_____

_____

17. Give an example of groupthink (in any setting).

_____

_____

_____

_____

18. Why should you document incidents of sexual harassment you may experience in the workplace?

_____

_____

_____

_____

MATCHING

Choose from the terms listed and match them with the best description. You may use an answer more than once.

_____ 19. An employee defends the improper behavior of another.

_____ 20. How we perceive a problem, situation, or action sometimes depends on our social and cultural background as much as our knowledge.

_____ 21. Can destabilize employee relations in a department

_____ 22. Prevent(s) effective rational problem solving

_____ 23. Promotes efficiency and equal sharing of resources

_____ 24. It is sometimes difficult to communicate verbally in the OR because of the background noise.

_____ 25. Waiting for the other person to finish the sentence before you speak

_____ 26. Can have a negative effect on our ability to understand and discuss a problem calmly

a. Good interdepartmental relations

b. Environmental barriers

c. Strong emotions

d. Perceptions

e. Bias

f. Lack of understanding

g. Social and cultural influences

h. Rumors

i. Respect for the other person

MULTIPLE CHOICE

Choose the best answer to complete the question or statement.

27. Professionalism is mainly determined by:
    a. The level of education and skills a person has
    b. One's ability to lead on a team
    c. The number of years a person has practiced his or her profession
    d. The individual's core values expressed in the workplace and community

28. The best person with whom to communicate a problem in the workplace is:
    a. Top management
    b. The head nurse
    c. A colleague who understands how you feel
    d. One who has the ability and authority to help solve the problem

29. The operating room requires its staff to work at a high level of mental, physical, and emotional strength. Because of this environment, the work may be:
    a. Different from most other professions
    b. Good
    c. Stressful
    d. Rehearsed

30. Cultural competence is:
    a. The ability to change one's belief system
    b. Being friendly with everyone
    c. Learning to speak another language
    d. Studying the cultural values of others

31. The model for good team relationships is:
    a. Respect for others
    b. A positive attitude
    c. Admiration by others
    d. The ability to change people's minds

32. When working with people with problem behaviors, one must remember to focus on the behavior and not the _____.
    a. Person
    b. Attitude
    c. Team
    d. Task

33. Chain of command is:
    a. An organized hierarchy of personnel positions and authority
    b. Usually only exhibited in the military
    c. Important only to management
    d. A list of personnel who have the authority to hire and fire

34. Verbal abuse is:
    a. Vulgar remarks to another person
    b. Violent public criticism demeaning another person
    c. Loud and abrasive comments or demands
    d. All of the above

35. Verbal abuse sometimes is built into the operating room _____.
    a. Culture
    b. Hierarchy
    c. Management
    d. Surgeons

36. Many people are reluctant to report abuse in the workplace for fear of:
    a. Losing friends
    b. Losing their job
    c. More abuse
    d. A bad employee review

37. _____ abuse takes place among staff members of equal rank and position.
    a. Lateral
    b. Verbal
    c. Vertical
    d. Physical

38. Sexual harassment is an extreme abuse of power in which a person engages in the following type(s) of behavior:
    a. Expects sexual favors in exchange for personal or professional gain
    b. Directs sexually explicit comments toward another
    c. Directs vulgar or sexual innuendoes at another
    d. All of the above

39. A _____ is a group of people who come together to reach a common goal or set of goals.
    a. Gang
    b. Team
    c. Professional
    d. None of the above

40. Setting team priorities requires a _____.
    a. Group
    b. Team
    c. Consensus
    d. Leader

41. Most role confusion is a result of poor _____.
    a. Teamwork
    b. Groupthink
    c. Attitude
    d. Communication

42. The goal of conflict resolution is to attempt to find a solution that is acceptable to all parties; this is called a _____ _____ solution.
    a. Win lose
    b. Win win
    c. Conflict resolution
    d. Open minded

43. A manager who makes most decisions with little or no input from the team is referred to as:
    a. Laissez-faire
    b. Democratic
    c. Experienced in groups
    d. Authoritarian

44. In the role of _____, the surgical technologist tutors the student and shares the duties of a scrubbed technologist.
    a. Team leader
    b. Preceptor
    c. Manager
    d. Instructor

CASE STUDIES

1. *The surgeon you are working with has been making personal comments about you that make you feel uncomfortable.*

   a. What should you do?

   b. Why is documentation so important in issues involving sexual harassment?

c. How do you know this is sexual harassment?

2. *Read the following scenario and answer the questions that follow.*

A surgical technologist is scrubbed on an exploratory laparotomy. The circulator and another staff member are chatting about a movie they both recently saw. The surgeon remains focused on the field. Suddenly there is unexpected severe hemorrhaging, and the patient's abdomen is rapidly filled with blood. The scrub is focused on putting appropriate clamps and an additional suction on the Mayo. Meanwhile, the circulator is unaware of the emergency. The scrub interrupts the circulator in his conversation and says loudly, "We need more sponges—you should pay better attention to the field."

After the patient has been taken to the postanesthesia care unit (PACU) and is stable, your circulator comes to you and states that you made him look "really bad" in front of the surgeons and the anesthesiologist.

a. Is the circulator's evaluation of the situation valid?

b. If the circulator has a valid point, how should the scrub respond?

c. How might this event effect the communication and teamwork between these two individuals in the future?

3 Law, Documentation, and Professional Ethics

Student's Name _____

KEY TERMS

Differentiate between the terms.

1. Negligence vs. intentional acts of harm: _____
   _____
   _____
   _____

2. Ethics vs. law: _____
   _____
   _____
   _____

3. Practice standard (guideline) vs. position statement: _____
   _____
   _____
   _____

4. Certification vs. licensure: _____
   _____
   _____
   _____

5. Malpractice vs. negligence: _____
   _____
   _____
   _____

6. Plaintiff vs. defendant: _____
   _____
   _____
   _____

7. Delegation vs. abandonment: _____
   _____
   _____
   _____

8. Practice acts vs. federal laws: _____

_____

_____

_____

9. Hospital policy vs. practice guidelines: _____

_____

_____

_____

10. State certification vs. state registration: _____

_____

_____

_____

11. Accountability vs. delegated task: _____

_____

_____

_____

SHORT ANSWERS

Provide a short answer for each question or statement.

12. Honoring the patient's privacy is a standard of conduct established by all health professions. What methods of communication are covered by the Health Privacy Act?

_____

_____

_____

_____

13. What are the requirements for the delegation of a task?

_____

_____

_____

_____

14. What is accountability, and how does it apply to the surgical technologist's role in the health care facility?

_____

_____

_____

_____

15. What does the Latin phrase *respondeat superior* mean?

_____

_____

_____

_____

16. Who is responsible when a delegated task results in patient harm or injury?

_____

_____

_____

_____

17. Define what negligence is in your own words.

_____

_____

_____

_____

18. Under what circumstances is it appropriate for a surgical technologist to refuse to take part in certain types of procedures?

_____

_____

_____

_____

MATCHING

Choose from the terms listed and match them with their most correct description. You may use the same answer more than once.

_____ 19. Decisions made by a court based on previous similar legal cases and decisions

_____ 20. Standards that meet or exceed the Joint Commission

_____ 21. State laws

_____ 22. Violation may result in disciplinary action by the facility

_____ 23. Regulations passed by agencies and departments of the government such as the Federal Drug Administration (FDA)

_____ 24. Practice acts

_____ 25. Logical, beneficial, and created by specialists within the organization

_____ 26. Signed into law by the governor

_____ 27. Based on precedence from previous cases

_____ 28. Rules established by the Environmental Protection Agency (EPA) for the handling of medical waste

a. Hospital policy

b. Statutes

c. Administrative law

d. Legal doctrines

11

MULTIPLE CHOICE

Choose the correct answers for the question or statement.

29. Example(s) of a sentinel event include (select all that are correct):
    a. The surgeon is habitually late for her cases
    b. A sponge was left inside the patient
    c. The pneumatic drill failed to work during a case
    d. The wrong drug was administered to the patient during surgery
    e. All of the above

30. The leading cause of patient injury in the operating room is:
    a. Falls
    b. Burns
    c. Surgical sponges left behind in the wound
    d. Abandonment

31. In an effort to decrease the number of wrong-site, wrong-patient injuries, the following protocol has been developed:
    a. QUICKCHECK
    b. VERIFY
    c. SURE-ID
    d. TIMEOUT

32. The correct care of surgical specimens (tissue or other) includes the following:
    a. Identification of the tissue during surgery
    b. Correct labeling of the specimen
    c. Correct method of containment
    d. Delivery of the specimen to the pathology department

33. HIPAA protects a patient's _____ and other health information through its privacy rule.
    a. Medical records
    b. Opinions
    c. Legal record including past convictions
    d. Constitutional rights

34. _____ represent(s) a permanent legal record of the patient's interaction with health care providers and services.
    a. Billing statement
    b. Entire patient record
    c. Discharge summary
    d. Signed consent

35. _____ is the process by which the attending practitioner explains the risks, benefits, and alternatives of the surgery to the patient.
    a. Health literacy
    b. Patient education
    c. Informed consent
    d. Discharge criteria

36. An incident report should include the following information (select all that are correct):
    a. The names of people who saw the incident
    b. The name of the patient's referring doctor
    c. Current medications prescribed to the patient
    d. Your opinion of what caused the incident
    e. What you did when the incident occurred
    f. Your evaluation of the patient's injuries
    g. Your opinion of how the incident should have been handled

CASE STUDIES

1. *Study the following incident and answer the questions:*

Surgical technologist "A" is required to scrub on the first case of the day. He is about to perform hand antisepsis when the circulating nurse notifies him that the case has been delayed. He decides to wait for the case while checking supplies for the next few cases. One of the nurses sees him and asks that he keep an eye on her patient who is waiting on a gurney in the hall. The patient is conscious. Another staff nurses approaches "A" and states that there is an emergency case and he is required to scrub as quickly as possible. "A" wheels the patient he has been observing close to the main desk. Although there is no one there at the time, he knows that there is a lot of foot traffic in that area and so he leaves the patient there. "A" hurries to the scrub sinks, performs hand antisepsis, and proceeds to his assigned room. Later, he is brought into the OR supervisor's office along with the nurse who asked him to watch her patient. He is told that the patient he was supposed to be watching earlier in the day had cardiac arrest and is now in the ICU in critical condition.

a. Who, if anyone, has been negligent?

b. Did anyone contribute to the patient's cardiac arrest?

c. If abandonment was committed, at what point did it occur?

d. Was the unit clerk at the front desk responsible for the patient?

e. What might be the consequences of this event?

2. *Study the following and answer the questions:*

Surgical technologist "B" has been working with several surgeons over a period of 6 months. One of the surgeons has been hinting that he will need a private tech to assist him at the office and in surgery and will begin interviewing for the position very soon. The position would carry a high salary and increased responsibilities over what "B" has been doing. Soon after the surgeon announces his news, "B" is assigned to scrub with him again. He states in confidence to "B" that he has only performed this type of surgery twice before. During the procedure, the surgeon makes a medical error by severing a major artery. The artery would have been easily identified and avoided by other surgeons in that specialty. Considerable blood is lost before the bleeding can be controlled. The patient's blood pressure drops precipitously, and the procedure is halted. As soon as the blood pressure begins to approach normal limits, the surgeon quickly finishes the case. The circulating nurse informs "B" that she intends to file an incident report and says that "B" must sign it also as a witness, or he can fill out another report on his own behalf. "B" decides that since the case ended with no *apparent* damage, he will not sign the report and does not intend to file another one.

a. Does this event require an incident report? Defend your answer.

b. Is this event considered an *incident* or a *near miss*?

c. If an incident report is written, is "B" obliged to sign it?

d. Since the event was an accident, is it considered negligence?

4 The Health Care Facility

Student's Name _____

SHORT ANSWERS

Provide a short answer for each question or statement.

1. Briefly explain what is meant by the following:

   a. Restricted area

   _____

   _____

   _____

   b. Unrestricted area

   _____

   _____

   _____

   c. Transition area

   _____

   _____

   _____

2. Briefly explain how the design (floor plan) of the operating room contributes to separation of restricted and unrestricted areas.

   _____

   _____

   _____

3. Containment is one way of controlling the rate of infection in the operating room. Briefly describe two examples of containment strategies in the OR.

   _____

   _____

   _____

4. Why do you suppose that traffic patterns in lounge areas in the operating room are difficult to control?

   _____

   _____

   _____

5. Why must the surfaces in the operating room be non-porous?

_____

_____

_____

6. How is air pressure in the operating room engineered for infection control?

_____

_____

_____

7. What is the influence of air temperature on patient care and safety?

_____

_____

_____

8. Why is it almost always unwise to skip the chain of command when reporting an incident or seeking information?

_____

_____

_____

9. The Joint Commission (JC) is a non-profit organization tasked with the accreditation of hospitals and health care facilities based on their compliance with a set of guidelines and protocols. Mark the following statements about accreditation "true" or "false."

a. **T**_____ **F**_____ Accreditation is mandatory for all hospitals and health care facilities.

b. **T**_____ **F**_____ An accredited health care facility qualifies for patient care reimbursement.

c. **T**_____ **F**_____ The JC is governed by state government officials.

d. **T**_____ **F**_____ The JC standards focus on quality care, safety, and protection.

e. **T**_____ **F**_____ JC standards are derived from state laws.

MATCHING

Match each term with the correct definition. Some terms may be used more than once.

10. _____ Lounge area

11. _____ Locker rooms

12. _____ Sub-sterile rooms between individual operating rooms

13. _____ Sterile core

14. _____ Surgical operations are performed here

15. _____ Sterile instruments are placed here during a procedure

16. _____ Used to hold instruments needed for immediate use during surgery

17. _____ Gases and suction are made available through this

18. _____ Patients are brought here just before surgery

19. _____ Used for receiving soiled sponges during surgery

20. _____ Must be maintained between 30% to 60%

a. Restricted area

b. Humidity in the OR

c. Semi-restricted area

d. Transition between unrestricted and semi-restricted area

e. Back table

f. Mayo stand/tray

g. Unrestricted area

h. Kick bucket

i. Procedure room

j. Inline system

k. Holding area

MULTIPLE CHOICE

Choose the best answer to complete the question or statement.

21. _____ is the economic use of time and energy to save unnecessary work, material resources, and time.
    a. Efficiency
    b. Engineering
    c. Environment
    d. Operations

22. _____ are physical routes for people and equipment in the health care facility that are designed to separate "clean" areas from "dirty" areas.
    a. Airflow
    b. Traffic patterns
    c. HEPA
    d. Front desks

23. The department is separated into three distinct areas:
    a. Restricted, semi-restricted, and clean
    b. Unrestricted, clean, and dirty
    c. Unrestricted, clean, and restricted
    d. Unrestricted, semi-restricted, and restricted

24. Only personnel in complete scrub attire, including hair cap, mask, and facial hair covering, are permitted in the _____ area.
    a. Restricted
    b. Unrestricted
    c. Semi-restricted
    d. None of the above

25. The _____ core contains clean and sterile equipment and supplies.
    a. Clean
    b. Sterile
    c. Equipment
    d. Dirty, soiled

26. The back table is a large stainless steel table on which all instruments, supplies, and equipment needed for surgery are arranged, except for those needed for:
    a. Immediate use
    b. Delivery of anesthesia
    c. Later in the case
    d. Suturing

PERSONNEL POLICY

Answer the following questions about personnel policy.

27. What is the difference between a job description and a job title?

_____

_____

_____

_____

28. Explain what *role confusion* is.

_____

_____

_____

29. In what ways does role confusion contribute to poor patient care?

_____

_____

_____

30. Why is it so important to ready and study the health care facility's personnel policy manual?

_____

_____

_____

5 The Patient

Student's Name _____

KEY TERMS

Provide the definition of each term.

1. Body image: _____

2. Developmental disability: _____

3. Infantilizing: _____

4. Sensory deficit: _____

5. Regression: _____

6. Patient-centered care: _____

7. Physiological: _____

8. Reflection: _____

9. Self-actualization: _____

SHORT ANSWERS

Provide a short answer for each question or statement.

10. Why is it important for a health care provider to examine his or her own core beliefs?

_____

_____

_____

_____

11. Why do many people feel a loss of control when they become a patient in a health facility?

_____

_____

_____

_____

12. How can you use your knowledge about developmental stages to communicate with the pediatric patient?

_____

_____

_____

_____

13. Explain the following statement: *The person is not the disease.*

_____

_____

_____

_____

14. Why are obese patients at risk for airway obstruction during surgery?

_____

_____

_____

_____

15. List some strategies for communicating with patients who have limited understanding of English.

_____

_____

_____

_____

_____

MATCHING

Match the developmental age with perceptions common to that age group. You may use an answer more than once.

16. _____ Prone to fantasy

17. _____ Very sensitive about body image

18. _____ Curious about how the body works

19. _____ Very frustrated with loss of autonomy

20. _____ Concrete thinkers, literal in their understanding of words

21. _____ Grateful for information about the environment and their procedure

a. Infant

b. Toddler

c. Preschooler

d. School age

e. Adolescents

MULTIPLE CHOICE

Choose the therapeutic communication which best fits the situation.

22. When communicating with young children your should try to:
    a. Treat them as small adults.
    b. Tell the truth using language they understand.
    c. Avoid the truth so they won't be frightened.
    d. Avoid answering questions about pain.

23. When caring for a blind patient you should:
    a. Speak loudly
    b. Avoid speaking about their blindness.
    c. Orient the patient to the environment verbally.
    d. Use hand signals to communicate.

24. When caring for the patient with a hearing deficit, you should:
    a. Find out what communication method the patient prefers
    b. Order an interpreter before you attempt to communicate
    c. Turn off the PA system in the OR
    d. Speak very loudly

25. When caring for the older patient, you should:
    a. Not assume the patient is cognitively impaired
    b. Treat the patient as you would a child
    c. Speak directly to the patient in a normal voice
    d. Clarify your communication as needed

1. *Read the following scenario and answer the questions.*

An 83-year-old patient has been brought to the operating room and is scheduled for a knee replacement in the room you are working in as an assistant circulator. The patient is wearing glasses and a hearing aid. The RN circulator greets the patient while you prepare the safety strap on the operating table. You and the RN circulator assist the patient in moving onto the operating table. The RN removes the patient's glasses and places them on the desk. You and the RN circulator continue to prepare for the surgery while keeping watch on the patient. The anesthesia provider enters the room. After the surgery is over and the patient has been taken back to his room on the ward, the ward nurse calls to ask about the patient's hearing aid and glasses. The patient does not have them, and they are not found in his room. Later in the day, the hearing aid is found in the laundry.

a. What could have happened to the hearing aid between the time the patient arrived in the operating room until his return to the ward?

b. What might have been the consequences for the patient if the hearing aid was not found?

c. How should the patient's glasses have been handled by the circulators (including yourself)?

d. Whose responsibility is it to take care of the glasses and hearing aid?

e. Should the patient have been allowed to wear the glasses and hearing aid to surgery? Explain your answer.

f. How do you think the patient may have reacted on finding out his glasses and hearing aid were missing?

2. *Read the following scenario and answer the questions.*

You are asked to transport a 44-year-old female patient from the ward to the operating room. You arrive on the ward and notify the head nurse that you are there to pick up the patient. You are directed to the correct room. When you arrive, the patient's family is with her. Everyone seems very worried, and the patient appears frightened. The patient's sister asks how long the procedure will take. You aren't sure, so you tell the family you do not know. The sister appears unhappy with the answer but does not press the question. She then states that she saw a program on TV in which a former patient describes being able to feel everything during his surgery, in spite of having received general anesthetic. You are not sure how to respond to this, so you say that the story was probably false and didn't happen. Finally, the patient's husband asks you if his wife will be in a lot of pain after the surgery. You don't want to worry the family, so you say that she probably won't have any. The patient has remained silent throughout the conversation.

a. What would be a better response to the sister's question about the length of the surgery?

b. Why are families generally concerned about the time length of a surgery?

23

c. What would be a better response to the sister's description of the TV show on conscious anesthesia?

d. What would be a better response to the husband's question about postoperative pain?

e. How do you think the total encounter with the family affected the patient?

f. How could you have practiced therapeutic communication with the patient, even in her silence?

6 Diagnostic and Assessment Procedures

Student's Name _____

Differentiate between the terms.

1. Acute vs. chronic illness: _____
   _____
   _____
   _____

2. Etiologic vs. idiopathic: _____
   _____
   _____
   _____

3. Morbidity vs. mortality: _____
   _____
   _____
   _____

4. Signs (of disease) vs. symptoms: _____
   _____
   _____
   _____

5. Prognosis vs. diagnosis: _____
   _____
   _____
   _____

6. Curative vs. palliative (treatment): _____
   _____
   _____
   _____

7. Invasive vs. noninvasive (procedure): _____
   _____
   _____
   _____

8. Hematocrit vs. hemoglobin (values): _____

_____

_____

_____

9. Benign vs. metastatic: _____

_____

_____

_____

10. Plain x-ray vs. fluoroscopy: _____

_____

_____

_____

SHORT ANSWERS

Provide a short answer for each question or statement.

11. The vital signs include:

_____

_____

_____

12. Why are vital signs measured?

_____

_____

_____

13. Explain the three- or four-point scale used to report the strength of the pulse, as well as the terminology used to describe the pulse.

_____

_____

_____

_____

_____

_____

14. Describe the technique for measuring the respiratory rate.

_____

_____

_____

15. Describe the technique of measuring the pulse using the correct terms.

_____

_____

_____

16. What problems are associated with the use of a simple digital (automatic) sphygmomanometer to measure blood pressure?

_____

_____

_____

17. How is respiratory rate measured?

_____

_____

_____

18. Blood pressure varies by age and is affected by various other normal physiological conditions, including:

_____

_____

_____

MATCHING

Match the blood pressure technique with its error. You may use the same answer more than once.

19. _____ Pressing the stethoscope too hard on the artery

20. _____ Cuff is too large for the patient

21. _____ Cuff is too small for the patient

22. _____ Failure to wait at least 2 minutes before retaking the blood pressure

23. _____ Cuff is deflated too quickly

24. _____ Cuff is deflated too slowly

25. _____ Air escapes from the cuff even when the valve is closed

26. _____ Stopping deflation and re-inflating the cuff

a. Faulty equipment

b. False high diastolic

c. False low diastolic

d. False low systolic

e. False high systolic

MATCHING

Match each term with the correct definition.

27. _____ Combines radiography with an image intensifier that is visible in normal lighting

28. _____ Is generated by high-frequency sound waves

29. _____ Uses radiofrequency signals and multiple magnetic fields to produce a high-definition image

30. _____ Uses the combined technologies of computed tomography and radioactive scanning

31. _____ X-ray and computer technologies are combined to produce high-contrast cross-sectional images

a. Computed tomography (CT)

b. Magnetic resonance imaging (MRI)

c. Fluoroscopy

d. Positron emission tomography (PET)

e. Ultrasound

MATCHING

32. _____ ABO system

33. _____ Complete blood count (CBC)

34. _____ Prothrombin time (PT)

35. _____ Platelet

36. _____ Arterial blood gas (ABG)

37. _____ Hematocrit

38. _____ Hemoglobin

39. _____ Pulse oximetry

a. Measures blood clotting time

b. Describes a person's blood type

c. Component that is necessary for blood clotting

d. Basic test used to evaluate the type and percentage of normal components in the blood

e. Measures blood oxygen saturation by spectrometry

f. Measured in grams of iron per deciliter

g. Specimen must be kept cold during transport

h. Measures percent of red blood cells by volume

MULTIPLE CHOICE

Choose the best answers to complete the question or statement. *You may choose more than one answer.*

40. The culture and sensitivity test is used to:
    a. Determine the presence of a foreign body in tissue
    b. Determine which antibiotics are effective against an infection
    c. Detect a specific infectious agent (microorganism)
    d. Detect the presence of pus in a wound

41. Excision is:
    a. The removal of a portion of tissue by making an incision
    b. The removal of tissue using a brush
    c. The removal of tissue using a needle
    d. Tissue fixation

42. A neoplasm:
    a. Is usually malignant
    b. Does not undergo histological change
    c. Is always benign
    d. Is any abnormal growth

43. Malignant tumors:
    a. Closely resemble the tissue of origin
    b. Release toxins that kill normal cells
    c. Capture nutrients from normal cells
    d. Take over the blood flow of normal tissues

44. Metastasis is:
    a. The spread of a benign tumor into other tissues
    b. The spread of cancer cells to distant locations in the body
    c. A tumor that exhibits organized growth patterns
    d. Often propagated by seed cells that break away from the tumor

45. Nuclear medicine:
    a. Is seldom practiced because of the danger of radioactivity
    b. Involves the use of gamma radiation
    c. Includes radiation therapy contained in pellets
    d. Is used to diagnose and treat malignancy

46. Magnetic resonance imaging (MRI) uses magnetic energy and therefore
    a. Can react with certain types of tattoos
    b. Is capable of drawing large metal objects into the machine
    c. Is mainly used to destroy tumors
    d. Requires the use of lead aprons

47. Which of the following statements about electrocar-diography (ECG) are true?
    a. Emits electrical signals that are picked up by the heart
    b. Produces a QRS wave
    c. Requires electrodes, which are placed on the chest and extremities
    d. Registers the conductive impulses of the heart

48. Which of the following statements about fluoroscopy are correct?
    a. Uses sound waves to form an image
    b. Requires the use of dye
    c. Allows x-ray images of the body to be observed in real time
    d. Requires a light box to view the images

CASE STUDIES

1. *Read the following scenario and answer the questions that follow.*

A surgical technologist who is new on the job is assigned to work in the outpatient clinic for minor procedures. Her role is to assist the circulator during the morning's work. The first patient arrives to have a skin lesion removed.

The circulator tells the surgical technologist to collect the equipment and forms necessary to take the patient's vital signs during the case.

The ST looks for a digital blood pressure cuff. Not finding one that is working, she obtains a manual sphygmomanometer and stethoscope. She cannot find a form for documenting the vital signs, so she takes a blank paper from the printer.

The case is about to begin. The ST explains to the patient that she will be taking the vital signs every 15 minutes.

The case begins with local infiltration of the lesion using lidocaine with epinephrine 1:200,000. After the infiltration, the ST begins to take the blood pressure reading. She cannot find the pulse at first because it is thready and weak. Finally she thinks she has located it and takes the reading. She records 145/95 on her paper. She records the pulse at 120 and respiration at 19. She knows that epinephrine can increase the pulse rate, so she is not concerned with the reading. The patient is slightly overweight, so the blood pressure reading also makes sense.

The ST continues to take the patient's vital signs over a 45-minute period. She skips the last reading because the skin incision has been closed. The patient is moved to a waiting area. The circulating nurse asks the ST for her documentation. When she sees it, she asks why the ST didn't use the appropriate form. The ST replies that she could not find one. The ST has recorded the vital signs as follows:

1- 145/95 pulse – 120 resp 19

2- 150/95 pulse – 120 resp 20

3- 135/90 pulse – 110 resp 12

She tells the circulator that the blood pressure changed as the anesthetic began to "wear off."

The circulator is somewhat disturbed at the scrub's explanations and documentation of the patient's vital signs. She asks the scrub why she did not record the middle blood pressure reading. The ST states that she didn't know it was required.

a. List all the errors made by the new ST in her new role.

b. Describe the correct procedure.

c. What could have been the patient care consequences of the errors?

7 Environmental Hazards

Student's Name _____

Differentiate between the terms.

1. Impedance (resistance) vs. conductivity: _____

   _____

   _____

   _____

2. Standard precautions vs. transmission-based precautions: _____

   _____

   _____

   _____

3. Technical risk vs. chemical risk: _____

   _____

   _____

   _____

4. Oxygen-enriched atmosphere (IEA) vs. pure oxygen: _____

   _____

   _____

   _____

5. Blood borne pathogen vs. airborne contamination: _____

   _____

   _____

   _____

6. Red bag (biohazard) waste vs. non-infectious waste: _____

   _____

   _____

   _____

7. True allergy vs. hypersensitivity: _____

   _____

   _____

   _____

8. Exertion vs. posture: _____

_____

_____

_____

9. Flammable vs. inflammable: _____

_____

_____

_____

10. Source of ignition vs. combustible material: _____

_____

_____

_____

SHORT ANSWERS

Provide a short answer for each question or statement.

11. What is the relationship between the concentration of oxygen and the speed of ignition?

_____

_____

_____

12. What do the elements of the fire triangle represent?

_____

_____

_____

13. What is a patient fire?

_____

_____

_____

14. Explain each RACE action during a structure fire.

   R _____

   A _____

   C _____

   E _____

15. Describe the function(s) of a gas regulator.

_____

_____

_____

16. Explain how compressed gas cylinders should be stored.

_____

_____

_____

17. We should never completely drain a medical gas tank because:

_____

_____

_____

18. What is an electrical ground? Why is it necessary for safety?

_____

_____

_____

19. What is the leading cause of hospital fires in the United States?

_____

_____

_____

MATCHING

Place the letter(s) corresponding to the correct answer.

20. A lead apron must be worn during procedures that use _____.

21. Lead aprons must be stored flat or hung to prevent _____.

22. Plastic and titanium objects are not affected by _____.

23. This is used after a needle stick injury: _____.

24. The minimum safe distance to avoid exposure to gamma radiation is

_____.

25. This is used to measure cumulative exposure to gamma rays: _____.

26. One of the components of a smoke plume is _____.

27. _____ is commonly used in skin prep solutions and represents a source of operating room fires.

a. Hydrogen cyanide

b. 6 feet

c. Cracking

d. Dosimeter

e. X-ray

f. Alcohol

g. MRI

h. PEP

MULTIPLE CHOICE

Choose the best answers to complete the question or statement.

28. The basic premise on which Standard Precautions are based is:
    a. Surgical patients are particularly prone to infection.
    b. All patients in the hospital pose a health risk to staff.
    c. Any patient can harbor a potentially infectious microorganism.
    d. We must use sterile technique even if the case is contaminated.

29. Which of the following statements is true regarding the high fire risk in the operating room?
    a. Oxygen is heavier than air and settles on the floor.
    b. Oxygen is lighter than air and tends to float above the anesthesia machine.
    c. Oxygen may become trapped in surgical drapes.
    d. When nitrous oxide decomposes in the presence of heat, oxygen molecules are produced, creating an oxygen-rich environment.

33

30. An environment that has a concentration of oxygen greater than 21% is called a(n):
    a. Oxygen-poor atmosphere
    b. Oxygen-enriched atmosphere
    c. Normal room air
    d. Oxidizing atmosphere

31. Which of the following is/are considered flammable?
    a. Endotracheal tubes
    b. Surgical drapes
    b. Fibrin glue
    c. All of the above

32. Which of the following are considered sources of ignition?
    a. Surgical drapes
    b. Lasers
    c. Chlorhexidine solutions
    d. Alcohol prepping solutions

33. During a colonoscopy, the potential for fire is high because of the high concentration of:
    a. Flammable drapes and equipment
    b. Oxygen
    c. Laser emissions
    d. Methane gas

34. On which of the following would you use a class A (water) fire extinguisher?
    a. Electrical fires
    b. Laser fires
    c. Flammable liquids
    d. Wood, paper, and cloth

35. Class B fire extinguishers recommended for operating room fires are also called _____ extinguishers.
    a. Bromochlorodifluoromethane
    b. Carbon dioxide
    c. Hydrogen peroxide
    d. Water

36. Compressed _____ is used as a power source for instruments, such as drills, saws, and other high-speed tools.
    a. Oxygen
    b. Argon
    c. Nitrogen
    d. Nitrous oxide

37. _____ is/are known to contain benzene, hydrogen cyanide, formaldehyde, blood fragments, and viruses.
    a. Peracetic acid
    b. Gas released from a sterilizer
    c. Smoke plumes
    d. HEPA filters

38. With regard to toxic chemicals in the operating room, which of the following statements is true?
    a. The cumulative effects can be much greater than the effects of any single exposure.
    b. Many of the chemicals are hazardous, but they usually produce only short-term effects.
    c. Guidelines for handling chemicals are designed to help in the development of risk strategies.
    d. Only the emergency department is required to maintain MSDS for chemicals.

39. The risk reduction strategy that is used after exposure to blood or other body fluids is called:
    a. PPE
    b. PEP
    c. PPP
    d. All of the above

40. _____ is a naturally occurring sap obtained from rubber trees.
    a. OPA
    b. Radiation
    c. Latex
    d. None of the above

41. _____ is the amount of physical effort needed to perform a task, such as moving an object.
    a. Posture
    b. Repetitive motion
    c. Exertion
    d. Contact stress

42. _____ is excessive direct pressure against a sharp edge or hard surface.
    a. Posture
    b. Repetitive motion
    c. Exertion
    d. Contact stress

43. When _____, keep the object close to your body.
    a. Lifting
    b. Pushing and pulling
    c. Bending
    d. Standing

44. When _____, place one foot behind the other; the back foot should be braced comfortably.
    a. Lifting
    b. Pushing and pulling
    c. Bending
    d. Standing

45. *Hands free* technique is:
    a. Putting the instruments on the Mayo tray during surgery and letting the surgeon take whatever instruments he or she needs
    b. A method of washing instruments in which only the machines touch them
    c. A self-retaining retractor system
    d. A method of passing the knife (scalpel) by putting it in a pan on the surgical field

46. *Transmission-based precautions* are used:
   a. When a patient is known or suspected to have a highly infectious disease
   b. When a staff member is known or suspected to have a highly infectious disease
   c. When a staff member has been exposed to HIV
   d. In emergency cases where the patient has not yet been identified

47. When using airborne transmission precautions:
   a. Staff members must wear masks at all times.
   b. The patient must wear a mask at all times.
   c. The patient and health care provider must wear a mask during surgery.
   d. The patient must wear a mask during transport.

CASE STUDIES

1. *Read the following scenario and answer the questions that follow.*

   Mrs. X has been admitted to the hospital for a breast biopsy with possible mastectomy. She is brought to the operating room, anesthetized using general anesthesia, and positioned for the surgery. The assistant circulator performs the patient skin prep using 70% alcohol iodophor paint. According to hospital policy, the extent of the prep must include the area required for a mastectomy—from chin to pubis. The surgeon enters the room during the prep and after gowning and gloving begins the patient draping procedure. After incising the skin, the surgeon requests the electrosurgical hand piece to coagulate a bleeding vessel. Within several seconds, the surgical site flares and the drapes are ignited. The fire spreads to the patient's abdomen in seconds. The scrub provides saline solution to put out the fire. The drapes are then removed to expose the extent of the injury. The patient sustains second-degree burns to 40 percent of her thorax and third-degree burns to her abdomen and pelvis. The operation is halted, and the burns are treated. The patient is taken to the ICU.

   a. What was the probable source of ignition?

   b. What was the fuel?

   c. What should have been done to prevent this accident?

d. Besides the patient burns, which will require more surgery and a lengthy hospital stay, what are the consequences for halting the original procedure and delay?

CRITICAL THINKING

1. The following quote from a lecture by Dr. B Boulanger at the University of Kentucky Medical School on safety in the operating room describes team member *focus* (distraction, preoccupation) as it relates to accidents in the operating room.

   "The OR team should be patient focused,
   • Not surgeon focused
   • Not work-flow focused
   • Not break focused
   • Not specialty focused
   • Not budget focused
   • Not Facebook focused!"

   Add 3 more similar points based on your knowledge of safety and negligence in the operating room.

2. What are the possible effects of communication failure on a culture of safety in the operating room? Provide examples to support your ideas.

8 Microbes and the Process of Infection

Student's Name _____

IMPORTANT TERMS

Finish the statements using the correct terms.

1. Microorganisms are everywhere in the environment. Most are harmless. Those that cause disease are said to be:

   _____

2. This type of microorganism is responsible for most human infections: _____

3. When we say an object or body tissue is *sterile*, what do we mean?_____

4. When an object or body tissue is no longer sterile, we say it is: _____

5. The process we use to kill all microorganisms on an object is called: _____

6. All body tissues are sterile except those that: _____

FILL IN THE BLANKS

Place the correct letter(s) corresponding to the missing word(s).

7. The dormant phase of a bacterium that is very difficult to kill is called a(n) _____.

8. When we grow a bacteria colony in the lab in order to perform tests it is called a(n) _____.

9. A specific test that identifies bacterial resistance to antibiotics is called a _____ and _____ test.

10. In order to clearly see bacteria under the microscope, we use a _____.

11. A type of bacteria found on normal skin is called _____.

12. The number of bacterial colonies on a surface is called the _____.

13. This sticky substance is produced by bacteria, allowing the cells to form an invisible barrier to destruction.

14. The proliferation of harmful bacteria in the body is called a(n) _____.

15. Bacteria commonly found in the large intestine are _____.

16. Malachite green is a type of _____.

a. Bioburden

b. Infection

c. Spore

d. Staphylococcus aureus

e. Sensitivity

f. Slime layer

g. Stain

h. Culture

i. Escherichia coli

j. Biofilm

SHORT ANSWER

Provide a real-life example of each type of microbial transmission.

17. Direct contact: _____

_____

18. Airborne transmission 1: _____

_____

19. Airborne transmission 2: _____

_____

20. Vector: _____

_____

21. Oral ingestion: _____

_____

SHORT ANSWERS

Provide a short answer for each question or statement.

22. Why is it important to identify microbes in the disease process?

_____

_____

23. What is a bacterial culture? Why do we perform this procedure?

_____

_____

24. How does the number of disease microbes at the site of entry relate to the process of infection?

_____

_____

25. List the tools for identifying microbes and give an example of each.

_____

_____

26. A surgical site infection may start as an abscess. What exactly is an abscess?

_____

_____

27. Why are bacteria the focus of study in disease microbiology?

_____

_____

MATCHING

Match the microbe with the correct definition.

28. _____ An organism lives on or within another organism (the host) and gains an advantage at the expense of that organism.

29. _____ One organism uses another to meet its physiological needs but causes no harm to the host.

30. _____ Nonpathogenic microbes (those that do not usually cause disease) that live in and on the body can become pathogenic under certain conditions.

31. _____ Each of the organisms benefits from their relationship in the environment.

a. Commensalism

b. Mutualism

c. Parasitism

d. Opportunistic organisms

MATCHING

Match the microbe with its characteristics. You may use the same answer more than once.

32. _____ Streptococcus, staphylococcus, meningococcus

33. _____ Anaerobes cannot live in the presence of oxygen

34. _____ Causes Aspergillus fumigatus, which invades the airways and causes vascular thrombosis

35. _____ Causes tuberculosis

36. _____ Requires water to survive; may have many intermediate hosts

37. _____ Replicates by invading another microbe cell

38. _____ Causes malaria

39. _____ Causes Clostridium difficile

40. _____ Causes polio and tetanus

41. _____ Resistant to all means of sterilization normally used in the health care setting

42. _____ Capable of transforming normal cells into cancerous cells

43. _____ Causes Creutzfeldt-Jakob disease

44. _____ Causes rabies

a. Bacteria

b. Virus

c. Prion

d. Fungus

e. Protozoa

MULTIPLE CHOICE

Select the best answer to complete the question or statement about disease transmission.

45. Disease-causing microorganisms are described as:
    a. Pathogenic
    b. Fomites
    c. Vectors
    d. Resistant

46. Harmful bacteria can be transmitted on dry airborne particles called:
    a. Aerosol droplets
    b. Aerosol vapor
    c. Contaminated dust
    d. Droplet nuclei

47. Bacteria can remain suspended in air as moist particles called:
    a. Droplet nuclei
    b. Aerosol droplets
    c. Droplet bacteria
    d. Contaminated droplets

48. Physical contact between tissue and an infectious microorganism is called:
    a. Contact transmission
    b. Direct contact
    c. Cell contamination
    d. Direct infection

49. The non-living object that transfers bacteria from one surface to another is called a:
   a. Vector
   b. Biofilm
   c. Dry nuclei
   d. Fomite

50. A person may become infected by bacteria in food that is eaten. This process of transmission is called:
   a. Digestion
   b. Ingestion
   c. Involution
   d. Digression

51. Insects and rodents that transmit infection are called:
   a. Parasites
   b. Animal transmitters
   c. Vectors
   d. Fomites

52. Not all contact with harmful microorganisms leads to an infection. Certain conditions must be favorable for the microorganism to gain entry to the body and proliferate. There must be (select all letters that apply):
   a. An entry site available
   b. A spore present
   c. Sufficient numbers of microbes
   d. An exit site
   e. No immunity
   f. Nutrients for the microbe
   g. Correct pH for the microbe
   h. Moisture

MULTIPLE CHOICE

Select the best answer to complete the question or statement about the phases of an infection.

53. In the _____ phase, symptoms begin to appear.
   a. Incubation
   b. Prodromal
   c. Acute
   d. Convalescence

54. In the _____ phase, the organism is at its most potent.
   a. Incubation
   b. Prodromal
   c. Acute
   d. Convalescence

55. In the _____ phase, the pathogens actively replicate.
   a. Incubation
   b. Prodromal
   c. Acute
   d. Convalescence

56. During the _____ phase, proliferation of the infectious organism slows and symptoms subside.
   a. Incubation
   b. Prodromal
   c. Acute
   d. Convalescence

MULTIPLE CHOICE

Select the best answer for each question regarding the process of infection.

57. The prion diseases are very significant in the surgical setting because
   a. They spread rapidly.
   b. All surgical patients are at risk.
   c. It is impossible to know who is a carrier.
   d. They are resistant to all usual methods of destruction.

58. Skin and mucous membranes are considered the first line of defense against disease because:
   a. Skin can be sterilized using disinfectants.
   b. Once the skin is broken, microbes can enter.
   c. Skin contains many blood vessels.
   d. Skin is very strong.

59. Which surgical wound is associated with the highest risk of infection in the postoperative patient?
   a. Clean
   b. Clean-contaminated
   c. Contaminated
   d. All of the above

60. The cardinal signs of inflammation are:
   a. Heat, redness, pain, swelling
   b. Pus, pain, redness, swelling
   c. Heat, pus, fever, pain
   d. Both A & C

61. Surgical site infection begins when a pathogenic or nonpathogenic microorganism colonizes sterile tissues. This can be caused by:
   a. Contamination of the tissues, such as a ruptured bowel or a traumatic wound caused by a foreign object
   b. External contamination of the wound during convalescence
   c. Poor surgical technique
   d. All of the above

40

62. Bacteria require basic elemental nutrients, *except*:
   a. Oxygen
   b. Sulfur
   c. Water
   d. Carbon

63. _____ exists from the time of birth.
   a. Innate immunity
   b. Adaptive immunity

64. _____ is conferred through exposure to a specific substance or microbe called an *antigen*.
   a. Innate immunity
   b. Adaptive immunity

65. _____ develops when the body receives specific disease antibodies from an outside source.
   a. Active immunity
   b. Passive immunity
   c. Vaccination
   d. Hypersensitivity

66. _____ is a process mediated by the immune system.
   a. True allergy
   b. Passive
   c. Vaccines
   d. Hypersensitivity

67. In certain diseases, the body does not recognize "self." This is known as:
   a. True allergy
   b. Autoimmunity
   c. Vaccines
   d. Hypersensitivity

68. There are two types of true allergic reactions:
   a. Immediate and reaction
   b. Reaction and delayed
   c. Delayed and immediate
   d. Immediate and true

CASE STUDIES

1. *Read the following scenario and answer the questions based on your knowledge of classification of surgical wounds.*

   You are scheduled for trauma call, and you get called in for a patient who was performing in a rodeo. He fell off his horse and is being admitted for an open fracture of the femur.

   a. How would this case be classified?

   b. What is this patient's risk for infection?

   c. If the wound was not open and the patient was admitted for a femoral fracture, how would the wound be classified?

9 The Principles and Practice of Aseptic Technique

Student's Name _____

KEY TERMS

Differentiate between the terms.

1. Antiseptic vs. disinfectant: _____

_____

_____

_____

2. Sterile field vs. surgical wound: _____

_____

_____

_____

3. Aseptic technique: _____

_____

_____

_____

4. Sterile vs. contaminated: _____

_____

_____

_____

5. Sterilize vs. disinfect: _____

_____

_____

_____

6. Scrubbed (sterile) personnel vs. nonsterile personnel: _____

_____

_____

_____

7. Resident bacteria vs. transient bacteria: _____

_____

_____

_____

8. Routine hand washing vs. traditional surgical scrub: _____

_____

_____

_____

SHORT ANSWERS

Fill in the blank for each question or statement regarding surgical attire.

9. A scrub suit must not be worn so tight as to cause _____ .

10. All surgical attire is made of fabric that sheds little or no lint to prevent _____

_____ .

11. Masks must be worn in all restricted areas of the operating room. They should not be worn dangling around the neck *at any time* because _____

_____ .

12. Surgical staff lockers are heavily laden with _____

_____ .

13. Home laundered head caps are not sanctioned by any infection control agency because _____

_____

_____ .

14. The scrub top should fit close to the body to prevent _____

_____

_____ .

15. The head cap or cover is donned before putting on a surgical top to prevent _____

_____ .

16. Eyeglasses or goggles worn during surgery must cover not only the eyes but also the _____ .

17. A surgical mask must be worn in _____ areas of the operating room.

18. The surgical mask is designed to prevent the release of _____ from the wearer's _____. The inside of the mask is therefore heavily laden with _____. This is why it should not be worn dangling:

_____ .

MATCHING

Match each statement with the correct term. You may use the same answer more than once.

19. _____ The application of an approved antiseptic to all surfaces of the arms, hands, and fingers

20. _____ A process meant to reduce the number of microorganisms on the skin to an absolute minimum using antiseptic soap, water, and a scrub sponge

21. _____ Should be timed or the strokes counted

22. _____ Ethyl or isopropyl alcohol combined with skin emollients

23. _____ Should be used only when no soil is visible on the hands

24. _____ Sponges must be sterile

a. Traditional surgical scrub

b. Surgical rub (antisepsis)

c. Routine hand washing

d. Hand rub antiseptic

MULTIPLE CHOICE

Select the best answer to the question or statement. There may be more than one answer per question.

25. The edge of a sterile wrapper:
    a. Should not be handled
    b. Is usually sticky
    c. Is protected from contamination
    d. Is not considered sterile

26. After an item has been sterilized, its sterility is maintained by:
    a. Keeping it in storage no longer than 30 days
    b. Preventing events that might contaminate it.
    c. Decontamination
    d. Keeping it in storage until the expiry date

27. The ethical and professional motivation that regulates a professional's behavior regarding disease transmission is known as:
    a. Tort
    b. Surgical law
    c. Surgical conscience
    d. Asepsis

28. A scrub suit must be changed if it:
    a. Is contaminated by blood or body fluid
    b. Comes in contact with the patient
    c. Comes in contact with any nonsterile item
    d. Has been worn for more than 5 hours.

29. When distributing a sterile solution to the scrub:
    a. It is necessary to pour the entire contents of the container at once.
    b. It is safe to replace the cap carefully so that more can be poured later.
    c. There is no way to protect the lip of the container.
    d. The circulator must pour the solution at least 24 inches away from the basin.

30. At the end of the shift, the surgical technologist may place the scrub suit in his or her locker if:
    a. It is unsoiled.
    b. It does not appear to be blood stained.
    c. The surgical technologist has worked less than 8 hours in it.
    d. The surgical technologist must never place the scrub suit in his or her locker at the end of a shift.

31. When changing from street clothes to a scrub suit for entering the operating room, the surgical technologist puts on which of the following items first?
    a. Scrub pants
    b. Shoe covers
    c. Scrub shirt
    d. Head covering

32. The term for the area under the fingernails is:
    a. Sublingual
    b. Subungual
    c. Buccal
    d. Ungual

33. The sterile gown is considered sterile:
    a. From the knees to the neck
    b. From the knees to the waist
    c. From chest to table height of the sterile field
    d. In the back as long as it is a wrap-around gown

34. The surgical scrub extends to:
    a. 2 inches above the elbows
    b. The elbows
    c. Just below the elbows
    d. The top of the shoulder

35. When sterile supplies have been opened, the sterile setup is vulnerable to contamination. Once the sterile supplies have been opened (select all that apply):
    a. They remain sterile for 1 hour.
    b. You must tape the OR door closed.
    c. They remain sterile for 2 hours.
    d. They must be continuously monitored to ensure sterility.

36. _____ is a way of making decisions and acting on proven methods.
    a. Evidence-based practice
    b. Surgical conscience
    c. Aseptic technique
    d. Academic research

37. _____ occurs when the surgeon's gloved hand accidentally touches the nonsterile edge of the surgical drape.
    a. Contamination
    b. A surgical error
    c. Antisepsis
    d. Aseptic technique

38. A sterile table (one draped with sterile covers) is sterile:
    a. From the top of the table to 3 inches below
    b. From the top of the table to 5 inches below
    c. At table height only
    d. From the top of the table to 3 inches below in front only

39. Items wrapped in _____ are best delivered directly to the scrub by grasping the top edges of the wrapper and peeling the wrapper apart to reveal the sterile item.
    a. Sterile wrap
    b. Sealed pouches
    c. Sealed wrap
    d. Original packages

40. When holding and opening a sterile package, the correct order of opening the flaps of the wrapper is:
    a. The side farthest away, the right and left, then the side closest to you
    b. The side closest to you, the right and left, then the side farthest away from you
    c. The right and left side, then the side farthest away from you, followed by the side closest to you
    d. If there is an addition sterile wrap underneath (the item is double wrapped), it does not matter.

TRUE OR FALSE

Answer the following questions about personnel hygiene "true" or "false."

41. **T____ F____** Frequent use of surgical hand antiseptic can dry the skin, resulting in small cracks that can become infected.

42. **T____ F____** Perioperative staff should keep the nails trimmed to ½ inch.

43. **T____ F____** A clean tee shirt can be worn under the scrub top as long as it doesn't show.

44. **T____ F____** Perioperative staff may wear nail polish as long as it is a neutral color.

45. **T____ F____** Jewelry can be worn by perioperative staff as long as it is covered with tape.

46. **T____ F____** Tattoos on exposed areas of the body are never allowed because they retain bacteria.

47. **T____ F____** Surgical personnel who harbor a skin infection or have open cuts can work in surgery as long as the area is covered with a bandage or tape.

CASE STUDIES

1. *Answer the following questions about evidence-based practice.*

    a. What is evidence-based practice?

b. Why is it so important in surgical practice?

c. Where does evidence-based practice come from?

d. Who is responsible for ensuring that only evidence-based practices are used?

CRITICAL THINKING

Surgeons who operate in several facilities may bring their own instruments for use in surgery. Sometimes the instruments are brought in already wrapped and sterilized. However, rules for aseptic technique require that instruments brought in from outside be opened, re-wrapped, and re-sterilized in the facility where the surgery takes place. Provide the rationale for this rule of aseptic technique. Note that there are a number of different reasons for this.

10 Decontamination, Sterilization, and Disinfection

Student's Name _____

_____

Differentiate between the terms.

1. Antiseptic vs. disinfectant: _____

    _____

    _____

    _____

2. Biofilm vs. bioburden: _____

    _____

    _____

    _____

3. Personal protective equipment (PPE) vs. scrub attire: _____

    _____

    _____

    _____

4. Prion vs. virus: _____

    _____

    _____

    _____

5. Ultrasonic cleaner vs. washer/sterilizer: _____

    _____

    _____

    _____

6. Cleaning vs. disinfection: _____

    _____

    _____

    _____

7. Reprocessing vs. sterilization: _____

    _____

    _____

    _____

8. Terminal decontamination vs. terminal cleaning: _____

_____

_____

_____

MULTIPLE CHOICE

Choose the best answer to complete the question.

9. The Spaulding system differentiates methods of sterilization for an item based on:
   a. Risk of infection
   b. What it is made of
   c. Whether or not it is used in the clinic
   d. How quickly it is needed

10. Critical/high risk items are those that contact:
    a. Sterile tissues
    b. Mucous membranes
    c. Skin
    d. Open wounds

11. Semi-critical/intermediate risk items come in contact with:
    a. Intact skin
    b. Vascular system
    c. Subcutaneous tissue
    d. Non-intact skin

12. Non-critical/low risk items come in contact with:
    a. Non-intact skin
    b. Mucous membranes
    c. Intact skin
    d. Semi-critical items

MATCHING

Match the Spaulding classification with the device. You may use the same answer more than once.

13. _____ Blood pressure cuff

14. _____ Hypodermic needle

15. _____ Operating room table

16. _____ Urinary catheter

17. _____ Stethoscope

18. _____ Oral thermometer

19. _____ Eye surgery instruments

20. _____ Transport gurney

21. _____ Anesthesia mask

a. Critical

b. Semi-critical

c. Non-critical

SHORT ANSWER AND MULTIPLE CHOICE

22. List the steps of reprocessing surgical instruments in order, starting at the point of use.

   a. _____

   b. _____

   c. _____

   d. _____

   e. _____

   f. _____

   g. _____

23. At the point of use after surgery is completed, the instruments are sorted and placed in basins. Heavier instruments are placed on the (a) _____ to prevent damage to (b) _____ instruments. Sharps are placed in a (c) _____. Water used to soak the instruments during surgery is (d) _____ to prevent (e) _____. All instruments and equipment are transported to the (f) _____ on a (g) _____ cart. Appropriate attire for work in the decontamination area includes _____, _____, _____, _____, _____, and _____.

24. The ultrasonic cleaner removes tissue debris and:

    a. Also sterilizes the instruments, including biofilm

    b. Does not sterilize the instruments and may not release biofilm

    c. Is performed with hot water and detergent

    d. Should be cleaned once per week using chlorhexidine

25. After decontamination, stainless steel instruments are brought to the _____, where they are sorted, _____ for damage, and prepared for sterilization. Instruments are placed in trays with _____ bottoms in order to allow _____.

26. Which of the following statements is *not* true regarding the use of peel pouches?
    a. Items wrapped in peel pouches must not be placed inside an instrument tray.
    b. Double pouches are unnecessary and may prevent sterilization of the item.
    c. The item in the pouch should clear the seal by at least 1 inch.
    d. Peel pouches are intended for items such as bone rongeurs, rasps, and multiple instruments.

27. The bacteria used as a biological indicator in steam sterilization are:
    a. Bacillus subtilis
    b. Geobacillus subtilis
    c. Geographillus stearothermohilus
    d. Geobacillus stearothermophilus

28. Biological monitoring should be performed:
    a. Whenever implants are sterilized
    b. On each load of goods for sterilization
    c. Once per month
    d. Once per day

29. Chemical monitoring proves that:
    a. The item is sterile.
    b. The item is safe to use for implantation.
    c. The parameters for sterilization were met during the process.
    d. The chemical is positive.

30. Items are wrapped before steam and EO sterilization in order to:
    a. Maintain sterility for 1 month
    b. Maintain sterility for 60 days
    c. Maintain sterility for 1 year
    d. Maintain sterility until an event occurs to contaminate the item

31. Implants must not be sterilized just before use in a "flash" sterilizer because:
    a. There is not enough time to run thorough biological testing.
    b. The item will be too hot.
    c. The item may be contaminated as it is transferred to the sterile field.
    d. There is no way to remove an unwrapped item from the sterilization tray.

32. The DART test is performed to:
    a. Detect pockets of concentrated steam
    b. Measure the quality of steam
    c. Detect air pockets
    d. Detect the moisture content in the sterilizer

TRUE OR FALSE

Answer the following questions about ethylene oxide (EO) sterilization "true" or "false."

33. **T_____ F_____** EO sterilization is commonly used because it is a rapid process.

34. **T_____ F_____** Items processed in EO require aeration in a designated area of the workroom.

35. **T_____ F_____** In order to reduce the amount of time of aeration of an item sterilized by EO, it is permissible to rinse it in sterile water before use.

36. **T_____ F_____** EO is highly toxic to the respiratory system.

37. **T_____ F_____** We can minimize staff exposure to EO by aerating goods inside the sterilizer.

CASE STUDY

1. *Read the following scenario and answer the questions.*

    You have scrubbed into your first case of the day. While preparing the instrument sets and supplies, you discover the following:
    • There is water in one of the basins that was wrapped.
    • A chemical indicator wrapped with a single instrument has not changed color.
    • There is moisture on the instruments in the set you need to prepare.
    • One of the hemostatic clamps has dried blood and tissue debris in the box lock.

    a. Explain what you should do immediately before the surgeons and patients arrive.

    b. Explain the probable cause of each problem and how it should have been prevented.

2. *Read the following case study and answer the questions about CJD that follow.*

Some microbes encountered in the environment cannot be destroyed by conventional means. An example is the microbe that causes Creutzfeldt-Jakob disease, which can be transmitted on neurosurgical instruments.

Another disease that is caused not by microbes but by reprocessing methods is TASS (toxic anterior segment syndrome) which may result in blindness.

a. What are prions?

b. What causes CJD?

c. Why is CJD a concern with regard to sterilization methods?

d. What is TASS? What are the AAMI guidelines to prevent TASS?

51

11 Surgical Instruments

Student's Name _____

KEY TERMS

Provide the definition for each term.

1. Metal alloy: _____
   _____
   _____

2. Scissoring: _____
   _____
   _____

3. Sizer: _____
   _____
   _____

4. Tungston carbide insert: _____
   _____
   _____

5. Annodizing: _____
   _____
   _____

6. One-piece scalpel: _____
   _____
   _____

7. Single action (ronguer): _____
   _____
   _____

8. Double action (ronguer): _____
   _____
   _____

9. Bevel: _____
   _____
   _____

10. Partial occlusion: _____

_____

_____

LABELING

Label the following diagram of a locking clamp.

11. _____

12. _____

13. _____

14. _____

15. _____

MATCHING

Match each instrument type with its classification. You may use the same answer more than once.

16. _____ Scalpel (knife)

17. _____ Hemostat

18. _____ Ronguer

19. _____ Tenaculum

20. _____ Osteotome

21. _____ Caliper

22. _____ Depth gauge

23. _____ Bougie

24. _____ Needle holder

25. _____ Thumb forceps

26. _____ Speculum

27. _____ Bone clamp

28. _____ Elevator

29. _____ Snare

a. Cutting

b. Clamping and occluding

c. Grasping and holding

d. Suturing

e. Dilating

f. Measuring

g. Stapling

h. Retracting

i. Suction

MATCHING

Match each Bard Parker knife handle with the correct blade. You may use the same answer more than once, and there may be more than one appropriate answer for each instance.

30. _____ #23   a. #3

31. _____ #10   b. #3 L

32. _____ #11   c. #7

33. _____ #12   d. #4

34. _____ #15   e. #4 L

35. _____ #20   f. #9

36. _____ #27

37. _____ #28

38. _____ #25

SHORT ANSWERS

39. *Safety first* is a priority that is emphasized throughout this textbook. Briefly state several ways that injury to team members *can be prevented* as instruments are passed and handled during a surgical procedure. Focus on safety only.

_____

_____

_____

_____

MATCHING

Match the tissue type with its characteristics.

40. _____ Tends to fragment when clamped; few blood vessels; slippery; lobular in structure; toothed instruments are used

41. _____ Highly vascular; delicate; can break apart when injured; must be handled carefully

42. _____ Resilient; strong; manipulation is by traction

43. _____ Occurs in fibers and bundles; slow to regain function when severed; usually moved aside rather than severed during surgery

44. _____ Very strong in healthy individuals; elastic; normally not cut with scissors during surgery

45. _____ Fine membrane; easily punctured; handled with smooth (not toothed) instruments only

46. _____ Resilient and strong; fibrous; elastic

47. _____ Slippery; strong; stringy; few blood vessels; handled with toothed instruments

a. Bone

b. Skin

c. Spleen, liver

d. Serosa

e. Muscle

f. Ligament

g. Tendon

h. Adipose (fat)

48. *Briefly describe the following classifications of surgical instruments. Be sure to include the materials of which they are made and the purposes for which they are used.*

   a. Surgical-grade instruments

   _____

   _____

   _____

   _____

   b. Floor-grade instruments

   _____

   _____

   _____

   _____

   c. Bright (or mirror) finish instruments

   _____

   _____

   _____

   _____

   d. Satin finish instruments

   _____

   _____

   _____

   _____

   e. Ebony finish instruments

   _____

   _____

   _____

   _____

12 Perioperative Pharmacology

Student's Name _____

KEY TERMS

Differentiate between the terms.

1. Concentration vs. volume: _____

_____

_____

2. Proprietary name vs. generic name: _____

_____

_____

3. Prescription drug vs. OTC drug: _____

_____

_____

4. Antibiotic vs. disinfectant: _____

_____

_____

5. Drug schedule vs. pregnancy category: _____

_____

_____

6. Dosage format vs. dosage: _____

_____

_____

7. Route of administration vs. dosage format: _____

_____

_____

8. Solution vs. tincture: _____

_____

_____

9. Contrast medium vs. stain: _____

_____

_____

10. Onset vs. peak: _____

_____

_____

11. Intravenous vs. topical: _____

_____

_____

12. Therapeutic window vs. toxic level: _____

_____

_____

13. Deca- vs. deci-: _____

_____

_____

14. International units vs. metric system: _____

_____

_____

15. Insulin syringe vs. tuberculin syringe: _____

_____

_____

16. Tampering vs. dispensing: _____

_____

_____

17. Ampule vs. vial: _____

_____

_____

18. Needle gauge vs. length: _____

_____

_____

SHORT ANSWERS

Provide answers for each question or statement about drug regulation.

19. The Joint Commission (JC) requires health care organizations to develop policies that agree with state laws (called *practice acts*). These regulate who may handle drugs and in what circumstances. *List* and *define* the activities concerned with handling drugs as covered by the state practice acts.

a. _____

_____

_____

b. _____

_____

_____

c. _____

_____

_____

d. _____

_____

_____

20. The Food and Drug Administration (FDA) maintains strict regulatory control on devices and substances used on or in the body. What are the organization's main duties with regard to public safety?

_____

_____

_____

_____

21. What is the meaning and significance of the *USP* label on drugs and medical devices?

_____

_____

_____

_____

22. What is a *controlled substance*? What agency of the federal government regulates controlled substances?

_____

_____

_____

MATCHING

Match each element of a drug label or package insert with its meaning.

23. The therapeutic amount to be administered

24. The patent name of the drug

25. A quantity of drug to be taken per unit of time

26. The name assigned to the drug by the USAN

27. The correct method(s) of drug administration

28. The regulated purpose of the drug

29. This can be traced in case the drug must be recalled for safety reasons

30. The date beyond which the drug must not be administered

31. A scannable label that verifies that a drug is not counterfeit

a. Dose

b. Expiration date

c. Generic name

d. Dosage

e. Proprietary (trade) name

f. Bar code

g. Lot number

h. Drug route

i. Indication

58

MULTIPLE CHOICE

Select the best single answer for each question about the drug process.

32. The *drug (medication) process* is:
   a. The methods and actions used by health care personnel to prepare, manage, transfer, and deliver a drug to the patient
   b. The methods used by pharmacists and nurses to mix drugs
   c. The action of a drug in the body.
   d. Laws that govern the prescribing and administration of drugs

33. In surgery, a drug prescription can be given as:
   a. The order on the surgeon's preference card
   b. A standing order
   c. A verbal order
   d. All of the above

34. The order for a drug can be transmitted by:
   a. Email
   b. Telephone
   c. Fax
   d. A & C only
   e. Verbally
   f. A, B, C, & E

35. A standing order is one that:
   a. Remains in effect until the patient leaves the hospital
   b. Remains in effect until the registered nurse changes it
   c. Remains in effect for 1 year
   d. Remains in effect until the prescriber changes it

36. Drug selection is a critical step in the medication process because:
   a. The registered nurse can be sued
   b. Drugs may have similar labels and names that sound alike
   c. It usually results in patient injury
   d. The surgical technologist is required to validate the selection

37. When medications are required on the surgical field, they should:
   a. All be distributed at the start of the case
   b. Be distributed at the time they are needed
   c. Be discarded during a change of personnel, such as a lunch break
   d. Be distributed just ahead of the time they will be needed

38. The surgical technologist is responsible for:
   a. Only drugs on the sterile field
   b. All drugs and solutions on the sterile field
   c. Only drugs that are administered to the patient during the surgery
   d. Only those drugs that are labeled on the surgical field

39. When labeling drugs on the sterile field, the minimum information required on the label is
   a. Date of preparation, name of drug, and strength of drug
   b. Date of distribution, name of drug, dosage, and route
   c. Date of preparation, name of drug, dosage, and expiration date
   d. Name of drug, strength of drug, and concentration of drug

40. The drug process requires that the surgical technologist and registered nurse:
   a. Together acknowledge the name of the drug, dosage strength, concentration, and maximum dose limit
   b. Should trust each other so the ST can distribute a drug when the nurse is unable to participate
   c. Identify the name of the drug only.
   d. Recite the 7 rights of a drug before transferring it to the sterile field.

SHORT ANSWER

41. List the seven drug rights and define them.

   a. _____

   b. _____

   c. _____

   d. _____

   e. _____

   f. _____

   g. _____

MATCHING

Match each measurement with the correct name and number. An answer may be used twice.

42. _____ = 1,000 meters

43. _____ = 1,000 grams

44. _____ = 1/1000 of a gram

45. _____ = 1/1000 of a liter

46. _____ = 5/1000 of a liter

47. _____ = 0.1 (one tenth)

48. _____ = 0.01 (one hundredth)

49. _____ = 0.001 (one thousandth)

50. _____ = 1 cubic centimeter

a. 5 *milli*liters

b. Deci

c. 1 *milli*gram

d. Centi

e. 1 *kilo*gram

f. Milli

g. 1 *kilo*meter

h. 1 *milli*liter

MATCHING

Match the route of administration with the dosage form. You may use the same answer more than once.

51. _____ Sublingual

52. _____ Intravenous

53. _____ Vaginal

54. _____ Intraosseous (IO)

55. _____ Subcutaneous (SQ)

56. _____ Intradermal (ID)

57. _____ Intramuscular (IM)

58. _____ Buccal

59. _____ Nasal

60. _____ Intraspinal

a. Parenteral

b. Oral

c. Topical

FILL IN THE BLANK

61. When drawing up a drug from an ampule, a _____ needle should be used.

62. A high alert drug is _____
_____ .

63. High alert drugs common in the surgical environment include (list each drug):

    a. _____

    b. _____

    c. _____

    d. _____

64. Blood products must be stored at a temperature range between _____ and _____ .

65. Blood and blood products must be used within _____ minutes/hours after withdrawal from cold storage.

66. Define the following and give an example:

a. Active hemostat _____

_____

b. Mechanical hemostatic agent _____

_____

c. Flowable hemostatic agent _____

_____

d. Anticoagulant drug _____

_____

e. Coagulant drug _____

_____

f. Vasoconstricting drug _____

_____

MATCHING

Match the phrases or sentences with the best answer concerning anesthetics.

67. _____ Reverses the effects of an opiate

68. _____ *Category* of drugs that causes rapid loss of consciousness, sensation, and autonomic reflexes; used for induction

69. _____ Used to relieve mild and moderate pain

70. _____ Describes a drug whose effect depends on the quantity administered

71. _____ Formulated and administered as a gas

72. _____ A drug given during specific cardiac emergencies to decrease the work of the heart

73. _____ Formulated as a liquid; administered as a gas

74. _____ Protects staff from exposure to anesthetic gases

75. _____ Category of drugs that alter the perception of pain; used as an analgesic

76. _____ Interferes with normal muscle cell depolarization

77. _____ Category of drug that induces drowsiness and depresses consciousness

78. _____ Produces dissociative anesthesia

a. Nitrous oxide

b. Barbiturate

c. Opiate

d. Scavenging system

e. Ketamine

f. Volatile anesthetic

g. Dose dependent

h. Neuromuscular blocking agent

i. Naloxone

j. Intravenous sedative

k. Morphine

l. Non-opiate analgesic

MULTIPLE CHOICE

Select the best answer to each question on local anesthetics

79. Local anesthetics are sometimes combined with epinephrine in order to:
    a. Prevent infection
    b. Increase the strength of the anesthetic
    c. Lengthen the peak action of the anesthetic
    d. Shorten the peak action of the anesthetic

80. The safe maximum dose of any local anesthetic depends on:
    a. The condition of the patient including age and weight
    b. What is written in the PDR
    c. The amount ordered by the surgeon
    d. The amount ordered by the anesthetist

81. Local infiltration of an anesthetic is:
    a. Injection of a blood vessel at the operative site
    b. Injecting the drug into the subarachnoids pace
    c. Administration of a bolus drug
    d. None of the above

82. Intravenous administration of epinepherine:
    a. Is frequently required during plastic surgery
    b. Is required during uncontrolled hemorrhage
    c. Can be fatal
    d. Is given to counteract the effects of an opiate.

CRITICAL THINKING EXERCISE

The operating room environment is complex in many ways. One of the complexities involves the way drugs are ordered, dispensed, handed over to scrubbed personnel, and handed over to the surgeon for administration. The following statements about the drug process describe tasks and events that routinely occur in the operating room. How does each situation affect or cause specific drug errors? Provide one or more errors that can be attributed to the situation described. Be specific.

1. Surgical personnel use complex medications requiring mixing and dilution of drugs using a variety of devices.

2. Surgical personnel routinely transfer medications from one container and deliver devices to others for administration to the patient.

3. Standard guidelines require all drugs to be relabeled on the surgical field. This involves handwriting at least some of the required information on a small label. Scrubbed personnel often use a skin marker that can smear and be washed over with blood or other fluids.

4. Surgical cases are often scheduled back to back with pressure to open up a case and set up quickly in order to maintain the surgical schedule.

5. The intraoperative environment is often noisy with the sounds of equipment, music, and talking.

6. Some drugs used during surgery are time sensitive. That is, they must be administered within a specified time limit after they are dispensed to the surgical field.

13 Anesthesia and Physiological Monitoring

Student's Name _____

Differentiate between the terms.

1. Sedation vs. coma: _____

_____

_____

2. Analgesia vs. anesthesia: _____

_____

_____

3. Anesthesia provider vs. anesthesia technician: _____

_____

_____

4. Endotracheal tube vs. nasotracheal airway: _____

_____

_____

5. Oxygenation vs. ventilation: _____

_____

_____

6. Perfusion vs. oxygen saturation: _____

_____

_____

7. Emergence vs. recovery: _____

_____

_____

8. Homeostasis vs. hemostasis: _____

_____

_____

9. Sedative vs. analgesic: _____

_____

_____

10. Sensation vs. awareness: _____

_____

_____

MATCHING

Match the physiological monitoring process with its purpose.

11. _____ Measures the level of neuromuscular blockade

12. _____ Measures blood pH

13. _____ Measures core temperature

14. _____ Measures the heart's rhythm, pitch, frequency, and intensity

15. _____ Monitors renal function

16. _____ Measures level of consciousness

17. _____ Measures cardiac output and central venous pressure

18. _____ Detects blood oxygen saturation

19. _____ Measures the levels of carbon dioxide produced during ventilation

20. _____ Measured by calculating the volume of irrigation fluid used during surgery, with total solution contained in the suction canisters

a. Bispectral index system

b. Capnography

c. Estimated blood loss

d. Peripheral nerve stimulation

e. Pulmonary artery catheter (PAC)

f. Pulse oximetry

g. Thermistor

h. Urinary output

i. Arterial blood gas

j. Transesophageal cardiac monitoring

SHORT ANSWERS

Fill in the blanks in this narrative on general anesthesia.

The process of general anesthesia includes different phases. During the first phase called (a) _____, the patient is given a fast acting drug that causes unconsciousness. Other drugs and gases are given to prolong uncon-

sciousness. That phase is called (b) _____. In order to maintain a *closed circuit* between the patient's respiratory system and the reservoir of anesthetic gas and oxygen, an airway is inserted. Two

common airways used according to the patient's requirements are the (c) _____ or

(d) _____. Two *stages* of general anesthesia are the most critical for preventing an airway emer-

gency. These are (e) _____ and (f) _____. Different types of airways are

used in the *semi-conscious* patient. The (g) _____ prevents the tongue or epiglottis from covering

the pharynx. However, if the patient has a mouth injury such as trauma to the lower face, a(n) (h) _____ is used. During the surgical plane of deep anesthesia, the patient receives a wide variety of adjunct drugs in order to

maintain (i) _____. Adjunct drugs and solutions may be required to provide muscle relaxation, improve cardiac tone, or balance blood pH. The *category* of drug administered to paralyze striated muscles during sur-

gery is called (j) _____. At the completion of surgery, the anesthetic agents are withdrawn and the

patient begins to regain consciousness. This initiates the (k) _____ phase of general anesthesia.

When the patient is stable, he or she is transported to the (l) _____.

MULTIPLE CHOICE

Provide the best answer to these statements about regional (local) anesthesia.

21. Regional anesthesia causes loss of sensation in a specific area of the body without alteration in:
    a. Heart rate
    b. Memory
    c. Which vital signs are monitored
    d. Consciousness

22. The maximum safe dose for each type of regional anesthetic is:
    a. The same for adult patients
    b. Dependent on the patient's weight, age, and medical history
    c. Dependent on the how well the drug works
    d. Monitored using the bispectral index system

23. The duration of effect of a regional anesthetic depends on:
    a. Its chemical formulation
    b. The patient's age
    c. The patient's level of consciousness
    d. The patient's level of sedation

24. When assisting the surgeon during local infiltration of anesthetic, the surgical technologist should:
    a. Use an 18 gauge and 19 gauge needle to inject the anesthetic
    b. Withdraw 10 mL of local anesthetic into two 20 mL syringes—one to have immediately and the other to use as needed
    c. Provide an Esmarch bandage as required
    d. Keep track of how much anesthetic has been injected throughout the case

MATCHING

Match each term with the correct definition.

25. _____ Regional anesthesia of a major nerve or group of nerves

26. _____ The spinal anesthetic blocks the nerves controlling the diaphragm and accessory breathing muscles

27. _____ Caused by a decreased cerebrospinal pressure usually related to a in the dura mater

28. _____ Intravenous regional anesthesia

29. _____ Anesthetic introduced into the caudal canal

30. _____ Anesthetic injected into the subarachnoid space

31. _____ Anesthetic injected into the epidural space through the lumbar interspace

a. Bier block

b. Spinal anesthesia

c. Postpsinal headache

d. Peripheral nerve block

e. Epidural anesthesia

f. Caudal anesthesia

g. Total spinal anesthesia

MULTIPLE CHOICE

Choose the best answer to complete the question or statement about surgical emergencies.

32. All health care workers in accredited facilities are required to be certified in CPR. The goal of CPR is:
    a. To restart the heart after a heart attack
    b. To restore cerebral circulation and function following a stroke
    c. To improve cardiac tone and oxygenation
    d. To restore ventilation, circulation, and oxygenation

33. Patients most likely to suffer an airway emergency in the operating room are those:
    a. With heavy musculature and fatty tissue in the throat
    b. Who cannot be positioned with the neck in hyperflexion (sniffing position)
    c. Who have a history of sleep apnea
    d. Who have a strong gag reflex related to excess tissue in the throat

34. Repeated unsuccessful attempts to intubate a patient may require a:
    a. Thoracotomy
    b. Tracheotomy
    c. Laryngectomy
    d. Cricoidectomy

35. Laryngospasm:
    a. Is relatively common in older patients
    b. Is only an emergency if the airway is obstructed
    c. Requires CPR
    d. Is related to the use of succinylcholine

36. Anaphylaxis is a true allergic reaction that may be exhibited by:
    a. Sudden loss of consciousness
    b. Sudden gagging
    c. Sudden dyspnea
    d. Sudden vomiting

37. A patient exhibiting anaphylaxis will likely be given:
    a. Epinephrine
    b. Succinylcholine
    c. Lorazepam
    d. Intravenous calcium

38. Hypovolemic shock occurs as a result of:
    a. Rapid severe loss of fluid from the body
    b. A cerebral stroke
    c. A myocardial infarction
    d. Severe tachycardia

39. Hypovolemic shock may be caused by:
    a. Severe hemorrhage
    b. Severe vomiting and diarrhea
    c. Severe burns
    d. All of the above

40. Hypovolemic shock can lead to:
    a. Multiple organ failure
    b. Gangrene
    c. Anaphylaxis
    d. Vasodilation

41. Malignant hyperthermia is a severe metabolic crisis that is precipitated by volatile anesthetics and:
    a. Succinylcholine
    b. Diazepam
    c. Epinephrine
    d. Neuroleptanalgesics

42. During a malignant hyperthermia crisis, the role of the surgical technologist is to:
    a. Remain sterile and protect the surgical wound
    b. Receive equipment and solutions for immediate body cooling
    c. As ordered, assist in closing the surgical wound to terminate the surgical procedure
    d. All of the above

43. Sudden severe hemorrhage during surgery may require which response by the scrubbed surgical technologist?
    a. The scrub might be asked to get blood from the blood bank.
    b. The scrub must help the surgeon clamp the bleeding vessel(s).
    c. The scrub must quickly prepare appropriate clamps, additional suction, or autotransfusion equipment as ordered.
    d. The scrub should expect additional staff to scrub in quickly and join the team.

44. Pulmonary embolism is prevented during surgery by:
    a. Ensuring that the patient has adequate oxygen during induction
    b. Asking the patient to take deep breaths before induction
    c. Applying a sequential compression device on the patient
    d. Keeping high risk patients in a reverse Trendelenberg position during the procedure

45. When the body is in a balanced physiological state, it is in:
    a. Hemostasis
    b. Balanced anesthesia
    c. Homeostasis
    d. Induction

46. Which of the following is *not* considered a protective reflex?
    a. Heartbeat
    b. Blinking
    c. Withdrawing from painful stimuli
    d. Shivering

Read the following scenario and answer the questions that follow.

A newly certified surgical technologist is in the first month of his job in a large hospital. Today he is preparing for a liver resection. During setup, the patient arrives. Meanwhile, the surgical technologist is occupied with the setup and concerned that he might not know all the instruments. However, he has followed the surgeon's preference card and with help from a colleague has arranged everything that is needed for the procedure. The surgeons have arrived, and the anesthesia provider has inserted two IV lines into the patient. He uses a barbiturate to induce the patient, who has a very large neck.

First minute: The anesthesia provider immediately places the patient in the sniffing position for intubation. His first attempt to intubate is unsuccessful. The circulating nurse is now assisting him, along with the anesthesia technologist.

Second minute: The anesthetist calls for a stylet and reaches for a different size endotracheal tube. The second attempt to intubate is unsuccessful. The patient is now having laryngospasms. His oxygen saturation is dropping quickly. The patient is dangerously hypoxic.

Third minute: The anesthetist tells the nurse to apply the BURP maneuver. Another nurse has entered the room and, seeing the situation, stands by with an emergency cricothyrotomy tray. The surgeon orders her to open it.

The surgical technologist receives the cricoidostomy tray and immediately places the knife, a clamp, and a tracheotomy tube on the sterile field; a second suction and suction catheter are also added. The surgeon is able to open the airway and insert the tube. He administers oxygen, and the patient is stabilized.

a. Why did the anesthetist put the patient in the sniffing position? What is the sniffing position?

b. Why did the AP need a stylet?

c. What is laryngospasm? Why did the patient's oxygen saturation drop?

d. How much time does the AP have to prevent brain damage in the event that no oxygen or very little is passing into the lungs?

e. Why did the AP require the BURP maneuver? What is it?

14 Postanesthesia Recovery

Student's Name _____

KEY TERMS

Differentiate between the terms.

1. Bronchospasm vs. laryngospasm: _____

    _____

    _____

2. Aspiration vs. respiration: _____

    _____

    _____

3. Hypoxia vs. anoxia: _____

    _____

    _____

4. Hypothermia vs. hyperthermia: _____

    _____

    _____

5. Hypoventilation vs. apnea: _____

    _____

    _____

    _____

SHORT ANSWERS

Provide a short answer for each question or statement.

6. When a patient is admitted to the PACU, the anesthesia care provider or registered nurse provides a handover to the PACU staff nurse. List five points that must be covered in the handover, plus a brief rationale explaining why each point is important, in your own words.

    a. _____

    _____

    b. _____

    _____

    c. _____

    _____

d. _____

_____

e. _____

_____

7. Any patient who is on a monitor during transport from the OR to the PACU must be accompanied by a(n)

_____ or _____ .

8. A focused assessment of the patient follows the general assessment. Why is a focused assessment performed?

_____

_____

9. The PACU is designed as an open floor plan with little furniture. Patients are taken to individual stations or bays for recovery. What is the purpose of the open floor plan?

_____

_____

10. PACU nurses are trained in critical care. Why is this necessary?

_____

_____

11. What is an ASA score, and why is it used in the PACU?

_____

_____

12. Patients who have undergone surgery of the thorax or abdomen may exhibit what respiratory problem. What is the reason for this?

_____

_____

13. Certain events that occur during surgery can result in persistent hypothermia in the recovery stage. Describe four such events.

a. _____

_____

b. _____

_____

c. _____

_____

d. _____

_____

MATCHING

Match each term related to postoperative monitoring with the correct system or function being monitored in the adult patient. You may use a letter more than once.

14. _____ Urinary output

15. _____ Facial expression

16. _____ Output of blood from drain

17. _____ Heart rate

18. _____ Patient ability to obey simple command

19. _____ Swelling at wound site

20. _____ Patient vocalization (e.g., moaning)

21. _____ Respiratory rate

22. _____ Oxygen saturation

23. _____ Protective reflexes

a. Core temperature

b. Pain

c. Wound assessment

d. Drains and catheters

e. Renal function

f. Neurologic function

g. Muscular response

h. Oxygen exchange

i. Peripheral circulation

j. Level of consciousness

MULTIPLE CHOICE

Choose the best answer to complete the question or statement.

24. When transporting a patient who is receiving oxygen by mask from the OR to the PACU, the tank must be:
    a. Placed next to the patient on the mattress
    b. Placed next to the patient at the foot of the mattress
    c. Held by the person accompanying the transport
    d. Secured in a tank holder attached to the gurney

25. Before transporting a patient who has been given a general anesthetic to the PACU:
    a. The patient's dentures must be in place
    b. The oropharyngeal airway must be removed
    c. The patient should be extubated
    d. The surgeon must sign the orders for pain medication

26. The surgical technologist may transport the patient unaccompanied to the PACU:
    a. According to hospital policy
    b. As long as he or she is certified
    c. As long as the anesthesia provider approves it
    d. As long as the patient is being monitored during transport

27. The Glasgow Coma Scale (GCS) measures the following parameters, except:
    a. Eye opening
    b. Verbal response
    c. Motor response
    d. Withdrawal from painful stimulus

28. The GCS is performed to evaluate:
    a. Brain death
    b. Neuromuscular response
    c. Reflexes
    d. Level of consciousness

29. Malignant hyperthermia is a condition that results in an extremely high core body temperature, cardiac dysrhythmia, tachypnea, hypoxia, and hypercarbia. What drug is administered to treat MH?
    a. Succinylcholine
    b. Demerol
    c. Dantrolene sodium
    d. Sodium chloride

30. Level of pain is evaluated in the adult patient using the following tools, except:
    a. Grimacing
    b. Core temperature
    c. Crying
    d. Heart rate

31. Pain level in the preverbal child is measured on the FLACC system by all of the following, except:
    a. Crying
    b. Facial expression
    c. Leg movement
    d. Eye opening

32. When a surgical patient is admitted to the PACU, the attending nurse needs to know the estimated or total blood loss that occurred during surgery. This is important because:
    a. It can have an effect on the patient's vital signs during recovery.
    b. It may be necessary to order blood for the patient.
    c. It may be necessary to order blood tests during recovery.
    d. All of the above

33. Hypothermia can produce physiological stress that may occur or persist during recovery. The affects of hypothermia include?
    a. Depression of the coagulation pathway
    b. Increased demand for oxygen by 400%
    c. Increased risk for adverse cardiac events
    d. All of the above

34. Which of the following is a false statement about malignant hyperthermia?
    a. It can be triggered by succinylcholine used to maintain cardiac tone.
    b. It causes cardiac dysrhythmia.
    c. It is a rare disease.
    d. It is potentially fatal.

35. Physiological objectives that are necessary to ensure patient safety outside the critical care unit are called:
    a. Apgar score
    b. Aldrete scale
    c. Discharge criteria
    d. Vital signs

CASE STUDIES

An ST has been hired in an ambulatory surgical day center that performs minor surgery using regional anesthesia and monitored IV sedation. The ST assists in procedures, prepares the equipment, and is responsible for equipment sterilization. It is a small facility, and on occasion the ST is asked to assist patients who are being discharged, especially toward the end of the work day. Today, the ST is asked to help with the discharge of the following two patients:

Patient 1 is a 70-year-old woman with a history of hip fracture in the past 6 months. She is in relatively good health but remains unsteady while walking. She uses a cane. She has met all discharge criteria. She is now waiting for a friend to pick her up and take her home. The friend is now 1 hour late. The ST has tried calling the friend several times but there is no answer. The patient is now anxious to get home and requests a taxi.

1. Can this patient be discharged to a routine taxi driver? If yes, how should this be done? If no, why not and what are the possible alternatives for the patient to get home?

2. If the patient is discharged and suffers a fall outside the facility, what is the responsibility of the facility staff, including the ST?

Patient 2 is a 50-year-old male who recently had a stroke and is now staying in a rehabilitation facility. He uses a wheelchair and has right side weakness of his arm and leg with difficulty speaking. He meets the discharge criteria. The driver from the rehab facility is waiting to take him back. However, the surgeon has not written the discharge orders and has left the facility.

1. What reasonable discharge plan and objectives can be made at this point?

2. The driver from the rehab facility states that he must leave to get another patient at another facility and will return. Will this work?

15 Death and Dying

Student's Name _____

KEY TERMS

Differentiate between the terms.

1. Heart-beating cadaver vs. non-heart-beating cadaver: _____

   _____

   _____

2. End of life vs. sudden death: _____

   _____

   _____

3. Direct cause of death vs. indirect cause of death: _____

   _____

   _____

4. A living will vs. a DNR: _____

   _____

   _____

5. DNAR vs. DNR: _____

   _____

   _____

6. Permission for recovery vs. required request law: _____

   _____

   _____

SHORT ANSWER

Provide a short answer for each question or statement.

7. When a physician pronounces the patient's entry into a dying state, the period is called _____.

8. In the United States, the medical and legal distinction for death is when _____ occurs.

9. In the United States, a manual called the International Classification of _____ is used to code all medical cases including intentional and unintentional trauma.

10. The cause of death is important to the family and community on an emotional level. It may also have implications

    for the recovery of _____.

Choose the best answer(s) to complete the question or statement about advance health care directives.

11. An *advance health care directive* is:
    a. Used in the event the person is unable to make decisions about health care
    b. A legal document in which a person states his or her wishes with regard to health care
    c. A category of documents regarding a person's health care wishes
    d. Deliberately vague to prevent conflict among family members

12. A person wishing to decline lifesaving efforts may sign a document that states:
    a. DNR
    b. DNAR
    c. Do not intubate
    d. Do not tube feed

13. A person may state in a legal document the exact nature of palliative care they want or do not accept. This document may be called:
    a. Right to die
    b. Palliative care rights
    c. DNR
    d. Living will
    e. Power of attorney
    f. All of the above

14. The _____ of death is considered by some to be too constricting and does not allow for individualism in the experience of death.
    a. Stage theory
    b. End of life theory
    c. Spiritual theory
    d. Psychological theory

15. _____ is the right of every individual to make decisions about how he or she lives and dies.
    a. DNR
    b. Advance directive
    c. Self-determination
    d. Living will

16. When no verifiable permission has been granted for organ donation by the patient, the _____ may act as a surrogate for the patient.
    a. Surgeon
    b. Family
    c. Chaplain
    d. Nurses

17. In the operating room, death is a(n) _____ event.
    a. Rare
    b. Occasional
    c. Weekly
    d. Daily

18. To qualify as a coroner's case, all of the following are mandatory for an autopsy, *except:*
    a. Death of an incarcerated individual
    b. Unwitnessed death
    c. Death after admission from the same facility
    d. Suicide

19. Organ recovery from a _____ cadaver is maintained on cardiopulmonary support to provide tissue perfusion.
    a. Non-heart-beating
    b. Heart-beating

20. Organ recovery from a _____ cadaver is restricted to tissue that does not require perfusion.
    a. Non-heart-beating
    b. Heart-beating

21. An _____ in effect in some states requires medical professionals to ask the family for permission to recover organs from the deceased.
    a. Required request law
    b. Permission request law
    c. Organ donation request law
    d. Permission to recover organs

22. Organ recovery protocols are:
    a. Determined by each health facility
    b. Determined by state law
    c. Determined by a non-profit organization
    d. Determined by county regulations

23. Organ recovery is usually performed by:
    a. A designated recovery team
    b. The team that is on call that day
    c. The emergency team
    d. Any team that is available.

CRITICAL THINKING EXERCISES

1. The ethics of dying and palliative care touch on issues that are often fraught with conflict. Consider the following:

   Families may have trouble deciding when to prolong life by supportive measures and when to discontinue them based on the suffering they might cause.

   a. What ethical issues are involved?

   b. What type(s) of advance care directive would resolve the ambiguity?

2. In the United States, organ donation and transplant is highly regulated by state and federal laws.

   a. Discuss several reasons why regulation is needed.

   b. What could be the consequences of not having enforceable regulations and laws?

   Note: Information on organ donation and transplant regulations can be found at http://www.organdonor.gov/legislation/.

16 Physics and Information Technology

Student's Name _____

KEY TERMS

Differentiate between the terms.

1. Amplitude vs. wavelength: _____

_____

_____

_____

2. Boiling point vs. freezing point: _____

_____

_____

_____

3. Conductivity vs. impedance: _____

_____

_____

_____

4. Element vs. molecule: _____

_____

_____

_____

5. Hot wire vs. ground wire: _____

_____

_____

_____

6. Reflection vs. refraction: _____

_____

_____

_____

SHORT ANSWERS

Provide a short answer for each question or statement.

7. The gaseous state of water is _____ .

8. The solid state of water is _____ .

9. The temperature at which a solid becomes a liquid is called the _____

    _____ .

10. Atoms are a discrete package of matter containing three main particles. These are the _____,

    _____, and _____.

11. The _____ has a positive charge. The _____ has no charge. The _____ has a negative charge and orbits the central particles.

12. Electromagnetic energy is propagated in the form of waves. Common forms of wave (electromagnetic) energy include:

    a. _____

    b. _____

    c. _____

    d. _____

13. Waves have predictable patterns and can be measured. The highest point of the wave is called a _____.

    The lowest point is called the _____.

14. When we *measure* the highest point of the wave, it is referred to as the _____.

15. The _____ is the *distance* from the highest point of one wave to the highest point of the next wave.

16. The number of waves that pass a point in 1 second is called the _____ of the waves.

17. When a wave reaches a substance it cannot pass through, it is _____ back.

MATCHING

Match each term with the correct definition as it applies to heat.

18. _____ Creates a current as the warm air rises and cool air falls

19. _____ The ability of a substance to conduct heat

20. _____ The transfer of heat from one substance to another by the natural movement of molecules, which sets other molecules in motion

21. _____ The displacement of cool air by warm air

a. Convection

b. Radiation

c. Thermal conductivity

d. Conduction

MULTIPLE CHOICE

Choose the best answer to complete the question or statement.

22. When an atom loses one of its electrons, the atom is left with a _____ charge.
    a. Positive
    b. Negative
    c. Neutral
    d. Alternating

23. The ability of a material to release free electrons is called:
    a. Static conductivity
    b. Impedance
    c. Conductivity
    d. Discharge

24. Free electrons are released and picked up within certain substances. This movement of electrons from one atom to another is called:
    a. Conduction
    b. Static
    c. Impedance
    d. Discharge

25. When electrical current meets resistance, it may be transformed into:
    a. Heat
    b. Vapor
    c. A proton
    d. An electron

26. A substance with low or no conductivity is called a(n):
    a. Resistor
    b. Voltage regulator
    c. Conduction resistor
    d. Insulator

27. As free electrons move through conductive material in a continuous path, the path is called an electrical:
    a. Path
    b. Flow
    c. Circuit
    d. Stream

28. The type of current that flows into a building from a power grid is a(n) _____ current.
    a. Alternating
    b. Alternative
    c. Direct
    d. Unidirectional

29. In the above electrical system, the power terminates at the:
    a. Receptacle
    b. Plug
    c. Wire
    d. Insulator

30. Three wires make up the pathway of an alternating current. The _____ wire is the power source from the power grid to the receptacle.
    a. Ground
    b. Blue
    c. Hot
    d. White

31. The _____ wire conducts electricity back to the grid.
    a. Neutral
    b. Hot
    c. Black
    d. Cold

32. The _____ wire picks up stray current and conducts it back to the grid and into the ground.
    a. Neutral
    b. Hot
    c. Red
    d. Ground

33. Electrical current will continue through a conductive material unless it meets resistance in the form of:
    a. Another conductive material
    b. Material that has low conductivity
    c. A reflection
    d. Material that has high conductivity

34. Electrical current will always seek a new path when it meets:
    a. Resistance
    b. The floor
    c. The body
    d. The circuit

FILL IN THE BLANK

Provide the best word to complete these sentences.

35. Laser light is composed of light rays that are lined up with peaks and troughs matching. This is called _____ light. In order to induce the light waves to line up, they are passed through a lasing _____.

36. Sound is created when an object vibrates and causes _____, which are propagated through a medium. Sound waves are measured like other wave energies. The _____ is called pitch. The amplitude is the _____ of the sound. Ultrasound uses sound waves that are _____ into a visual image.

37. The Doppler effect creates sounds that we perceive as high and low _____.

MATCHING

Match the term with the definition.

38. _____ Memory

a. Alphanumeric device for inputting data into the computer

39. _____ Motherboard

b. Also called RAM

40. _____ Drive

c. Data from a computer that has been reproduced in the form of a CD

41. _____ Monitor

d. The computer screen where data is viewed by the user

42. _____ Keyboard

e. Provides sound output from the computer

43. _____ Mouse

f. The primary circuits that run the computer

44. _____ Speakers

g. The user's steering component

45. _____ Hard copy

h. Internal or external device that stores the computer's data

CRITICAL THINKING

Based on what you know about electricity and electrical pathways, explain how a person can be electrocuted by touching an ungrounded circuit with bare hands.

17 Energy Sources in Surgery

Student's Name _____

KEY TERMS

Differentiate between the terms.

1. Active electrode vs. return electrode: _____

   _____

   _____

2. Alternating current (AC) vs. direct current (DC): _____

   _____

   _____

3. Amplification vs. frequency (of a wave): _____

   _____

   _____

4. Cauterization vs. electrosurgery: _____

   _____

   _____

5. Coagulum vs. eschar: _____

   _____

   _____

6. Monopolar circuit vs. bipolar circuit: _____

   _____

   _____

FILL IN THE BLANK

Fill the blanks with the correct words to complete the sentences.

7. The body reacts to electricity according to the voltage and frequency. High _____ is

   potentially more dangerous than low _____. High _____ is

   less dangerous than low _____.

8. The direct application of a heated instrument to tissue is called _____.

9. This is different from ESU, which uses _____ to cut and coagulate tissue.

10. The surgical technologist must be able to identify the components of the ESU system. The _____ is the contact point between the tissue and the flow of electrical energy generated by the ESU. This is attached to a handpiece often referred to as a "_____." The _____ is the source of power for the system and contains all the controls. The _____ (PRE) is placed close to the surgical wound site and captures the current from the _____ and returns it to the power unit. The simple name for this is the _____.

11. The original prototype of the ESU system was called the _____. This name is still used by some surgeons, although the original produced in the 1930s was very different and many more times dangerous than the ESU of today.

12. Two types of circuits are used in ESU. The _____ circuit does not require a dispersive electrode attached to the patient. The tip contains two contact points. Electricity flows from one _____ to the other without passing through the patient's _____.

13. In _____ circuit ESU, the electricity passes through the patient's body, is dispersed through the _____, and then returns to the power source.

14. Extended contact between the tissue and electrode tip results in the formation of _____. This can increase impendence and may cause _____.

MULTIPLE CHOICE

Select the best single answer to the following questions or statements.

15. Tissue fulguration uses:
    a. Pulsed application of electricity
    b. Low voltage electricity
    c. A thin beam of electricity
    d. Ultrasonic vibratioins

16. Electrosurgical vessel sealing uses bipolar energy, which creates:
    a. Eschar
    b. Pressure
    c. A weld in the tissue
    d. An incision

17. During surgery, the electrode pencil should be placed in a:
    a. Moist sponge
    b. Dry area
    c. Small basin
    d. Holster

18. During the use of monopolar ESU, the return electrode pad must be placed:
    a. Far away from the incision site to prevent the release of stray current
    b. Usually over the sacrum
    c. Close to the incision site to capture all current
    d. Usually over the abdomen

19. The power cord is attached to the drapes to prevent it from falling away from the surgical field. This is done with:
    a. A metal towel clip
    b. A metal clamp
    c. Any metal instrument
    d. None of the above

20. When the surgeon "buzzes" an instrument, he or she:
    a. Places a clamp over tissue and applies the ESU to the clamp
    b. Applies the ESU directly to tissue
    c. Applies bipolar electricity to a clamp
    d. Is violating OSHA regulations

21. Capacitative coupling occurs during endoscopic surgery when:
    a. There is a break in the insulation covering an instrument
    b. Current passes through the insulation and into adjacent tissue
    c. The active current leaks from the insulation
    d. All of the above

22. Direct coupling only occurs when:
    a. The active electrode or stray current comes in contact with another conductive instrument
    b. The electrical discharge at the inactive electrode couples with the active electrode
    c. The active electrode and other instruments compete for the circuit
    d. All of the above

23. Hazards associated with smoke plume are reduced by using:
    a. The normal suction device used for aspirating fluids in the surgical wound
    b. A specialized smoke evacuator
    c. HEPA filters in the room ventilation system
    d. None of the above

24. Ultrasonic energy is used to:
    a. Cut and coagulate tissue
    b. Coagulate tissue only
    c. Create coagulum that cuts through tissue
    d. Burn tissue

25. Examples of ultrasonic energy systems used during surgery include the:
    a. Harmonic scalpel
    b. Hemosure
    c. Sonisurge
    d. Sonisure scalpel

26. The ultrasonic device must be placed on a _____ directly after use.
    a. Dry towel to prevent conduction of electricity on the field
    b. Top drape
    c. Moist towel
    d. Dry sponge

27. During laser use, light waves are directed into a sealed chamber filled with:
    a. Nitrous oxide
    b. A laser liquid
    c. The lasing medium
    d. A lasing by-product

28. Two common types of lasers are the continuous wave laser and the:
    a. B-type wave laser
    b. Bypass wave laser
    c. Controlled wave laser
    d. Pulsed wave laser

29. The effect of the laser on tissue depends on:
    a. The power setting, laser frequency, and laser absorption
    b. The power setting, laser wavelength, and absorption quality of the tissue
    c. The power setting, absorption quality of the tissue, and temperature of the light
    d. The laser frequency, laser absorption, temperature of the tissue

30. One of the most important determinants of what kind of laser is used in a specific surgery is the:
    a. Absorption quality of the tissue
    b. Temperature of the laser
    c. Potential transformation of the tissue into a vapor
    d. Patient's allergies

31. Safety precautions are strictly observed when laser energy is in use. Among the most important is airway protection during head and neck surgery. The risks are related to:
    a. The use of high flow oxygen during these procedures
    b. The possibility of igniting flammable anesthetics
    c. The risk of the laser energy consuming available oxygen going to the patient
    d. The ignition of the endotracheal tube by the laser

32. What is the role of the surgical technologist during a patient fire?
    a. Immediately deliver saline or water to the surgical field
    b. Remain focused and follow the surgeon's orders
    c. Help extinguish the fire
    d. All of the above

33. When the ESU electrode tip touches tissue, electricity is _____, creating intense heat.
    a. Impeded
    b. Volted
    c. Coagulated
    d. Cut

34. In the _____ mode, the electrode is held above the tissue, without contact, and the air between the electrode and tissue acts as a conductor, allowing the high-voltage current to flow between the tissue and the electrode.
    a. Blended
    b. Cutting
    c. Desiccation
    d. Microbipolar cutting

35. _____ is therapy in which a probe is inserted into a tumor or tissue mass.
    a. Ultrasound
    b. Phacoemulsification
    c. Cryoablation
    d. Laser

36. When laser light is directed at a surface, which of the following will *not* occur?
    a. Absorption
    b. Coagulation
    c. Reflection
    d. Scattering

37. _____ is the use of an extremely cold instrument or substance to destroy tissue.
   a. Ultrasound
   b. Phacoemulsification
   c. Cryoablation
   d. Cryosurgery

38. _____ is created when electricity is transformed into mechanical energy generated by high-frequency vibrations and the focus on friction.
   a. Ultrasound
   b. Phacoemulsification
   c. Cryoablation
   d. Ultrasonic energy

39. _____ is performed by inserting a series of needle probes directly into the tumor under direct fluoroscopic imaging.
   a. Ultrasound
   b. Phacoemulsification
   c. Ablation
   d. Cryosurgery

CASE STUDIES

Read the following case studies and answer the questions based on your knowledge of patient safety when the ESU is used.

1. Your patient arrives in the preoperative holding area. His history and physical include an implanted electronic device (IED). Special considerations will be required for his elective surgery, because electrosurgery is planned during the procedure. What special precautions must be taken to keep this patient safe during surgery?

2. Your female patient is coming to surgery today, and your surgeon would like to use the laser during her procedure. What safety precautions will the operating room team need to understand and undertake before the laser is used for the patient's procedure?

18 Moving, Handling, and Positioning the Surgical Patient

Student's Name _____

SHORT ANSWERS

Provide a short answer for each question or statement.

1. Patient identification takes place many times during patient interaction with the health care facility. One way is by a unique identifier. Provide two examples of a unique identifier.

   _____

   _____

2. Another (different) method of identification is the:

   _____

3. When asking the patient his or her name, always use a closed-ended question. Provide an example of how to ask the patient's name using this method.

   _____

   _____

4. Describe five causes of skeletal injury among health care workers, including surgical staff.

   a. _____

   b. _____

   c. _____

   d. _____

   e. _____

5. When transporting the patient on a gurney, three pedal operations are available. Describe the action of each.

   _____

   _____

   _____

   _____

6. What is the purpose of the back board?

   _____

   _____

7. When pushing the gurney forward, you need to use the _____ setting.

8. When maneuvering the gurney in tight spaces, use the _____ setting. The setting is not used for travel.

9. A standard wheelchair can accommodate up to _____ pounds body weight.

10. When transporting a patient in a gurney or wheelchair, face forward except when _____ or

when _____.

MULTIPLE CHOICE

Select the best answer to these questions regarding the bariatric patient.

11. When moving and handling the obese patient, the objectives are to prevent injury and also provide the patient:
    a. Dignity
    b. Extra large blankets to prevent hypothermia
    c. With detailed information about his or her procedure
    d. Isolation from other patients in the environment

12. The obese patient may have comorbid conditions such as:
    a. Airway obstruction, severe allergies, diabetes
    b. Hypoxia, hypocapnea, hypotension
    c. Diabetes, poor peripheral circulation, pulmonary hypertension
    d. DVT, congenital heart defects, kidney disease

13. Special equipment required for the treatment of the obese patient include all but:
    a. Operating table capable of at least 500 lbs body weight
    b. Extra wide safety straps on gurneys, OR tables, and wheelchairs.
    c. Extra wide blood pressure cuffs
    d. Extra large stethoscopes

14. Patients in police custody in the health care setting may be required to:
    a. Stay quiet
    b. Undergo a test for tuberculosis before surgery
    c. Have all their belongings locked in the safe
    d. Be held in hard restraints

15. When transporting a child in a crib, it is important to:
    a. Never leave the child alone
    b. Take the top off the crib so the child can stand up
    c. Try to prevent the child from crying
    d. Travel as quickly as possible to decrease the amount of time spent in the crib

16. Unless it is contraindicated for safety (medical) reasons, the head of the gurney should be _____ during transport.
    a. Raised so the patient can see the environment
    b. Leveled to prevent others from seeing the patient
    c. Lowered to maintain the patient's blood pressure
    d. Raised to prevent cardiac arrest.

FILL IN THE BLANK

Fill in the correct word(s) to these statements about potential patient injury related to positioning.

17. The most common position resulting related to eye injury is _____. Continuous pressure on

tissue can result in a decubitus ulcer; This injury results in the breakdown of _____. Musculoskeletal injuries such as _____ can occur when joints are moved outside their normal range

of _____. Another common positioning injury is called _____. This

injury occurs when skin is pulled in one direction while deeper tissues are _____ in another.

MULTIPLE CHOICE

Choose the most correct answer to complete the question or statement.

18. When placing the patient in stirrups, it is necessary to:
    a. Position both legs at the same time
    b. Position one leg at a time
    c. Keep the patient's knees straight
    d. Dorsiflex the feet

19. A headrest that consists of pins that penetrate the patient's scalp and bone is the:
    a. Airplane headrest
    b. Gardner headrest
    c. Horseshoe headrest
    d. Doughnut headrest

Chapter **18** Moving, Handling, and Positioning the Surgical Patient

20. When positioning the pregnant patient, a foam wedge is placed:
    a. Under the right hip and flank
    b. Under the knees
    c. Under the left hip and flank
    d. Under both hips and flanks

21. A foam wedge is needed for the pregnant patient to:
    a. Release pressure on the lower back
    b. Release pressure on the vena cava
    c. Release pressure on the uterus
    d. Release pressure on the aorta

22. When the patient is shifted from supine to reverse Trendelenburg, the scrub must:
    a. Watch the patient's blood pressure on the monitor
    b. Notify the anesthesiologist of the change
    c. Remove all retractors from the wound
    d. Raise the Mayo stand

23. When cane stirrups are used, the foot straps should be positioned:
    a. Around the Achilles tendon and ankle
    b. Around the Achilles tendon and foot arch
    c. Above the Achilles tendon
    d. Over the Achilles tendon and ball of the foot

24. Another name for Allen stirrups is:
    a. Candy cane stirrups
    b. Fish fin stirrups
    c. Knee crutches
    d. Yellow fin stirrups

25. When placing the patient in lithotomy position:
    a. The table should be tilted to facilitate the positioning
    b. The arms should be at the patient's sides with the hands and wrists over the table break
    c. The shoulders should be padded to prevent pressure on the brachial plexus
    d. The hips should be rotated externally

26. Fowler's position may be used for:
    a. Perineal, knee, hip surgery
    b. Shoulder, breast, neuro surgery
    c. Back, neck, elbow surgery
    d. Maxillofacial, ear, mandible surgery

27. Lateral decubitus position is also called:
    a. Thoracic position
    b. Kidney position
    c. Flynn's position
    d. Sims position

28. When describing the lateral position, the terms "right" and "left" are used. These indicate which side is:
    a. The non-operative side
    b. The operative side

29. In the lateral position, the lower leg is:
    a. Flexed
    b. Straight
    c. Slightly flexed

30. In the lateral position, the safety strap is:
    a. Placed over the patient's hip
    b. Placed at the patient's waist
    c. Placed at the patient's knees
    d. Not needed

31. A vac pac positioner is also called a:
    a. Foam pack
    b. Foam triangle
    c. Air pack
    d. Bean bag

32. In the lateral position, a pad is placed:
    a. In the axilla
    b. Under the flank
    c. Below the axilla
    d. Above the axilla

33. In the prone position, the arms usually are positioned:
    a. At the patient's sides
    b. Laterally
    c. With the elbows flexed 90 degrees
    d. With the elbows flexed 180 degrees

34. In the prone position, gel rolls are placed:
    a. From the clavicle to the iliac crest
    b. From the clavicle to the mastoid bone
    c. From the iliac crest to the knees
    d. At the patient's sides to stabilize the position

35. The spinal table is fitted with a(n):
    a. Mirror so the patient can see himself during the procedure
    b. Padded perineal post
    c. Knee crutch on both sides
    d. Mirror so the anesthesia provider can observe the patient's head and neck

CASE STUDIES

1. Critical Thinking Exercise

   Read the scenario and answer the question.

   Surgery is scheduled for a patient requiring gastric banding at 17:00. This patient, Mr. X, is a 45-year-old male weighing 177 kilograms (390 lbs). He has been in the waiting area for 1 hour, and the team is ready to bring him into OR 2 for the procedure. Next door in OR 1, an emergency C-section is about to start. In OR 4 across the hall, a patient scheduled for a laparotomy earlier in the day is just now being brought in, as the surgery schedule is running behind.

   Circulating nurse A and the orderly bring Mr. X into OR 2. The circulator notes that the operating table in the room is a standard size. However, Mr. X's weight is just about within the limits of the table, so he proceeds with patient preparation on this table. Following an uneventful induction, prep, and draping, the procedure begins. Within 15 minutes, the surgeon calls for the table to be tilted for better exposure. Within moments, the patient begins sliding from the table. The team attempts to catch the patient but is unable to hold him. The patient slips from the table and falls to the floor. The team calls for help. Only a few other staff members are able to respond to the emergency. The patient suffers multiple fractures, including the skull and hip. The patient dies 3 days later as a result of irreversible shock.

   Provide an analysis of this scenario, detailing what factors contributed to the accident and what steps should have been taken to prevent the fall. Be specific in your analysis. Consider not only the problem of equipment but also safe positioning, staff responsibilities, and environmental factors.

2. *Read the following case study and answer the questions based on your knowledge of patient positioning and use of the operating room table.*

   You have been asked to set up the operating room for a procedure. Today your surgeon will perform an open thoracotomy in operating room 2. The surgeon has told the team that he will be using a posterolateral incision on the right side.

   a. In what position will the patient be placed?

Chapter **18** **Moving, Handling, and Positioning the Surgical Patient**

b. How will the arms be positioned?

c. Where will the gel pads be placed specifically?

d. How will the position be maintained during surgery?

19 | Surgical Skin Prep and Draping

Student's Name _____

LABELING

In the drawings below, use a colored pen or pencil to indicate the prep for the procedure listed.

1. Anterior head and neck

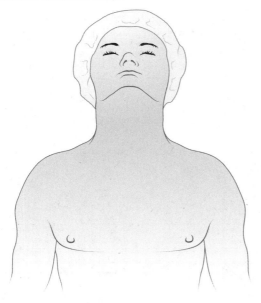

2. Anterior shoulder

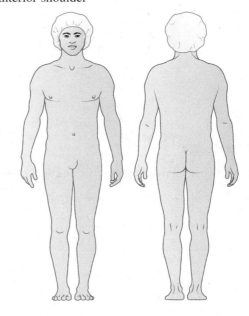

3. Back

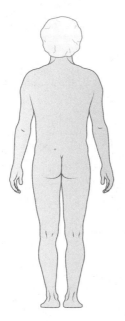

4. Abdomen

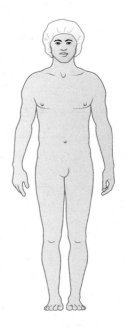

5. Inguinal area

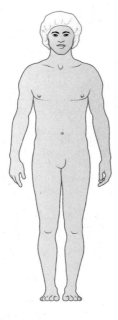

SHORT ANSWERS

Provide a short answer for each question or statement.

6. What is the purpose of the patient surgical skin prep?

_____

_____

_____

7. Which antiseptics are safe for use on the face?

_____

_____

_____

8. Which antiseptics are approved for use on the eye?

_____

_____

_____

9. Which antiseptics are safe for use on the mucous membrane?

_____

_____

_____

10. What is residual activity as it is applied to antiseptics?

_____

_____

_____

11. Why is the patient provided a hospital garment to wear during day (come and go) surgery?

_____

_____

_____

12. Under what circumstances is it necessary to wash the skin with antiseptic soap before applying skin prep paint?

_____

_____

_____

13. Why is pre-surgical skin marking performed?

_____

_____

_____

14. Explain the statement "There is no perfect skin antiseptic and no one solution for preventing SSI."

_____

_____

_____

15. When a tincture is used to prep the skin, it must be completely dry before drapes are applied. Why?

_____

_____

_____

16. When prepping a site that is potentially more contaminated than the surrounding area *within the prep boundary*, which is prepped first—the less contaminated area or the more contaminated area? Explain your reasoning. Provide examples.

_____

_____

_____

MULTIPLE CHOICE

Choose the best answer to complete the sentence or to answer the question:

17. When prepping the skin using alcohol-based products, it is critical that:
    a. The product is completely dry before applying drapes.
    b. Prep solution is prevented from pooling under the patient.
    c. The skin is checked for burns after the surgery.
    d. All of the above

18. Alcohol-based prep solution should not be used on:
    a. The ear or eye
    b. Mucous membranes
    c. The genitals
    d. Infants
    e. All of the above

19. Alcohol-based skin prep can easily wash off the surgical skin marking unless it is done with:
    a. A waterproof pen
    b. Crimson violet
    c. Venetian red
    d. Gentian violet

20. During a full body prep, it is important to:
    a. Prevent hypothermia
    b. Have enough supplies after you start
    c. Double glove
    d. Start draping when one prep area is dry

21. An autograft site is often prepped using:
    a. Mineral oil
    b. Clear prep solution
    c. Plain soap and water
    d. 15% betadine solution

22. The surgical prep for a craniotomy:
    a. Requires the head to be shaved
    b. May require the head to be shaved
    c. Requires the patient's hair to be braided
    d. Requires the use of metal pins to hold the hair away from the incision site

MATCHING

Match each term with the correct definition. Some terms may be used more than once.

23. _____ Sticky drape—one full side coated with adhesive

24. _____ Used in laser surgery

25. _____ Collects fluids, including blood from the surgical wound

26. _____ Waterproof sheet or area of the drape

27. _____ Has two tails

28. _____ Four towels are placed at the periphery of the surgical site

29. _____ Has a "window" in it for the incision

30. _____ Sticky drape—one edge coated with adhesive

a. Aluminum coated drape

b. Squaring the incision

c. Pocket or pouch drape

d. Incise drape

e. Towel drape

f. Fenestrated

g. Split drape

h. Impervious

CRITICAL THINKING

Provide the rationale (in your own words) for each of these rules of asepsis that apply to draping. Think about contamination of the prep site, contamination of the person(s) draping, and contamination of the drapes during draping. This exercise requires you to integrate what you learned about aseptic technique with draping principles and practice.

1. Handle drapes with as little movement as possible.

2. When placing a drape, do not touch the patient's skin or any other nonsterile surface.

3. After a drape is placed, do not shift it or move it.

4. Areas of the drape that fall below the level of the operating table are considered contaminated.

95

20 Case Planning and Intraoperative Routine

Student's Name _____

TRUE OR FALSE

Mark the statements about specimens "true" or "false."

1. T_____ F_____ Specimen containers should be labeled before the specimen is received.

2. T_____ F_____ Specimen labels should be placed on the container, not the lid.

3. T_____ F_____ All tissue specimens are transported in formalin (formaldehyde).

4. T_____ F_____ When transporting a specimen, the documentation should be placed inside the bag with the specimen.

5. T_____ F_____ Biopsy tissue which will undergo immediate frozen section must never be placed in formalin.

6. T_____ F_____ A foreign body removed from the patient should be wiped clean with a moist sponge and placed in a dry specimen container.

7. T_____ F_____ Lymph nodes that require immediate pathological examination are submitted in a dry container.

8. T_____ F_____ Muscle tissue for biopsy should be packed using an ice slush before transport.

9. T_____ F_____ Tissue retrieved from a patient for use in another patient requires registration with the FDA.

MATCHING

Match each term with the correct description.

10. _____ Removing a large portion of a tumor, but not all of it

11. _____ Separation of tissue without using sharp instruments

12. _____ Carefully separating anatomical structures by cutting with instruments, small firm sponges, or the fingers

13. _____ Refers to the removal of a limb or digit

14. _____ To constrict a vessel using a suture tie

15. _____ The joining of two hollow anatomical structures (vessels, ducts, tubes, or hollow organs) using sutures or surgical staples

16. _____ Using sharp surgical instruments such as a scalpel and scissors to cut away dead or devitalized tissue

17. _____ Bringing a tissue structure partially outside the body

18. _____ Separating tissue planes

19. _____ Removing tissue, usually a tumor, or other small lesion using cutting instruments or electrosurgery

20. _____ An undesirable pucker in skin as a result of poor suture placement

21. _____ In surgical terms, "bringing together" tissues by suturing or other means

a. Amputate

b. Anastomose

c. Approximate

d. Blunt dissection

e. Debridement

f. Dog ear

g. Debulk

h. Dissect

i. Elevate

j. Excise

k. Exteriorize

l. Ligate

96

MATCHING

Match each person with the correct role(s). You may use the same answer more than once.

22. _____ Unsterile team member

23. _____ Responsible for labeling the surgical specimen

24. _____ Adjusts the surgical lights as needed during the procedure

25. _____ Escorts the patient to the operating room from preop holding

26. _____ Opens the sterile supplies onto the sterile field as the room is being opened

27. _____ Performs the surgical scrub, and gowns and gloves himself or herself

28. _____ Involved in the TIMEOUT

29. _____ Responsible for maintaining a clean and orderly instrument table and sterile field

30. _____ Prepares and passes instruments during surgery

31. _____ Signs the surgical count sheet

32. _____ Performs the surgical count

33. _____ Documents the surgical procedure

34. _____ Looks for a missing sponge

35. _____ Directly responsible for identifying, receiving, and maintaining specimens on the surgical field

36. _____ Requests additional equipment as needed

37. _____ Directs the surgical team during an emergency

a. Scrubbed surgical technologist

b. Circulator

c. Surgeon

d. All team members

e. Scrubbed surgical technologist and circulator

MULTIPLE CHOICE

Choose the most correct answer to complete the question or statement.

38. Which of the following specimens might be sent to the pathologist on a Telfa sponge?
    a. A bullet
    b. Prostate from a transurethral resection of the prostate (TURP)
    c. Uterus and fallopian tubes
    d. Breast tissue for frozen section

39. Which of the following specimens must be sent to the pathologist dry?
    a. Colon polyps
    b. Bronchial washings
    c. Kidney stones
    d. Tonsils

40. A sympathetic nervous response that occurs when the bowel is not handled gently is called:
    a. Paralytic ileus
    b. Small bowel obstruction
    c. Ulcerative colitis
    d. Diverticulitis

41. _____ instruments are passed firmly.
    a. Ophthalmic surgery
    b. Orthopedic surgery
    c. Plastic surgery
    d. General surgery

42. Which sponge is used to prepare a sponge stick?
    a. Laparotomy
    b. 4 × 4
    c. Neuro surgical cotton
    d. Patty

43. Which type of sponge is used for blunt dissection?
    a. Kittner
    b. Neuro patty
    c. Cotton ball
    d. Laparotomy

44. Which type of sponge would be appropriate for "packing" the abdominal cavity?
   a. Kittner
   b. 4 × 4
   c. Laparotomy
   d. Neuro patties

45. Case planning combines knowledge of:
   a. Surgical procedure and surgical techniques
   b. Anatomy and pathology
   c. The patient's diagnosis
   d. The patient's prognosis

46. When opening packages sealed with tape, why should you break the tape rather than tear it?
   a. To prevent the outer wrapper from ripping, causing contamination
   b. So that you have to look at the tape to see whether it has changed color
   c. To prevent strike-through
   d. To reduce the amount of paper waste

47. Which of the following is *not* a recommendation for opening a case?
   a. Open the scrubbed surgical technologist's gown and gloves on a small table or Mayo stand.
   b. Never unwrap a heavy item by holding it in midair.
   c. Do not open small sterile items into the instrument tray.
   d. Open extra sutures, special equipment, and implants so that the surgeon does not have to wait for them during the procedure.

48. After the case has been opened, the surgical technologist's next immediate task is to:
   a. Load the knife blade
   b. Drape the Mayo stand
   c. Perform a surgical hand scrub
   d. Organize the instruments

49. Creating a continuous sterile field:
   a. Allows the surgeon to reach for instruments
   b. Contaminates the back table
   c. Saves steps and motion
   d. Uses up valuable space

50. After finishing the surgical scrub, which task is done next?
   a. Arrange towels, gowns, and gloves in order of use.
   b. Gown and glove self.
   c. Organize the knife and the instruments.
   d. Put all sponges in one location so you are ready to count.

51. The selection of suture material is almost always prescriptive, or:
   a. Written on the surgeon's case plan ahead of time
   b. Delayed until the surgeon can prescribe the type he or she wants
   c. Determined only after the surgeon has taken a look at the surgical wound
   d. Delayed until the surgeon has discussed surgical wound closure with the patient

52. If the count is incorrect:
   a. An x-ray is taken immediately
   b. The surgeon should not be bothered
   c. The surgeon is notified and the count is repeated
   d. The circulator should begin filling out an incident report

53. A retained item can cause patient injury from all of the following, *except*:
   a. Extended anesthesia time
   b. Infection
   c. Organ perforation
   d. Obstruction

54. Before the first count of the surgery, the scrub should:
   a. Do a preliminary count as a baseline
   b. Ensure there are enough sponges for the entire case
   c. Place all sponges and sharps in groups
   d. Place all sponges in a basin

55. After you scrub and as you first approach the pile of sterile equipment, do not move anything until:
   a. You have a plan
   b. You count the instruments
   c. You load the blade on the knife handle
   d. You move the drapes and put them in order

56. The surgeon's preference card:
   a. Is a legal document
   b. Is used to gather supplies for the procedure
   c. Cannot be relied on in most facilities
   d. Is rarely used in modern facilities

57. When opening sharps for a case, they should be:
   a. Opened into a large basin
   b. Opened on top of the drapes
   c. Distributed to the scrub just before surgery begins
   d. Ideally distributed directly to the scrub

58. According to law, who may take the surgical count?
   a. Anyone on the team
   b. Only the circulator and scrub
   c. Only a registered nurse circulator and scrub
   d. Only the surgeon, registered nurse, and scrub

59. The surgical count is taken in the following circumstances. Indicate all that apply:
    a. Before the first incision is made
    b. After the incision is made but before a body cavity is entered
    c. Before a joint capsule is closed
    d. Immediately before the closure of a body cavity
    e. When new supplies are distributed to the scrub
    f. When there is a question about a retrained item
    g. Before an x-ray is taken

60. What must be counted during the surgical count?
    a. Sponges and needles
    b. Instruments and their parts
    c. Stainless steel suture ends
    d. Aneurysm clips
    e. Anything that can be lost in the wound

SHORT ANSWER

Answer the following questions.

61. What is a "suture book"?

_____

_____

62. Who is responsible for ensuring that no item is left in a patient?

_____

_____

63. What is Universal Protocol (TIMEOUT)?

_____

_____

64. How can a needle stick be prevented in the operating room?

_____

_____

65. What methods can be used to prevent a tissue graft (such as a bone graft) from falling on the floor during surgery?

_____

_____

_____

_____

_____

CASE STUDIES

1. *Read the following case study and answer the questions.*

A 49-year-old female is admitted to the health care facility and scheduled for an open laparotomy with possible hysterectomy. The patient is 5 feet, 3 inches tall, 180 pounds, with a BMI of 31.9. After spending a short time in the holding area, the patient is brought into the OR by the circulating nurse. The scrub has begun setting up the case. She notes the patient's stature and requests extra clamps and sutures. The circulator states that she will get these after the case is under way.

After transferring the patient to the operating table and preparing the required documents, the nurse is ready to take a count with the scrub. All items are counted and recorded on the count sheet by the circulator.

The surgical procedure was started on time and is progressing well. The surgeon has decided to go ahead with the hysterectomy. The circulator has opened extra sponges onto the back table and waits for the scrub to count them with her. These are added to the count sheet. The scrub asks again for extra sutures. The circulator states that she will tell the nurse who is about to relieve her for a break. The relief nurse has come into the room and opens five extra suture packs onto the back table. Before these can be counted, the scrub distributes several to the surgeon. After the uterus has been removed, the surgeon announces he is ready to close. The first circulator has come back into the room just as closure is about to start.

According to policy, the circulator and scrub begin the count. One sponge and one suture needle are missing. The team finds the sponge in a basin, but the needle cannot be found. The surgeon continues to close the peritoneum. By the time skin closure has started, the needle has not been located. The patient is transported to the PACU and an x-ray is ordered there.

a. What *systematic* steps should be taken to find the missing needle?

b. What errors in standard practice do you notice in this case?

c. What standard practices should have been followed?

100

d. What steps should be taken by members of the team if the needle is not identified on the x-ray?

e. Why do you think the surgeon finished closing even when the needle was not found?

f. What do you believe will be the next steps if the needle *is* located on the x-ray taken in the PACU?

Student's Name _____

SHORT ANSWERS

Provide a short answer for each question or statement about the principles of surgical technique.

1. Signs of tissue dryness during surgery are:

    a. _____

    b. _____

    c. _____

2. When retracting tissue, it is necessary to use only the amount of pressure needed to _____

    _____

    _____ .

3. When irrigation is used during surgery, the scrub must keep track of the _____

    _____

    _____ .

4. Self-retaining retractors are always passed to the surgeon in which position?

    _____

    _____

5. Retraction using sharp skin hooks can cause _____

    _____

    _____ .

6. What is meant by the term *hemostasis*?

    _____

    _____

    _____

7. Pooling of blood in the surgical wound during healing may cause:

    a. _____

    b. _____

8. Surgical sponges are used for a variety of different reasons during surgery. Name three.

   a. _____

   b. _____

   c. _____

9. Autotransfusion is a way of salvaging the patient's blood during surgery. Describe briefly in your own words what the autotransfusion equipment does.

   _____

   _____

   _____

   _____

   _____

10. Sponge dissectors are used to perform _____ .

MATCHING

Match each term with the correct definition as it applies to implants and grafts.

11. _____ Tissue implanted in the patient removed from another person

12. _____ Any type of tissue replacement or device placed in the body

13. _____ Graft taken from beef origin

14. _____ Graft taken from pig tissue

15. _____ Tissue obtained from the patient's body and implanted in another site in the same patient

16. _____ Graft made up of more than one type of tissue

17. _____ Graft taken from an animal or synthetic source

18. _____ Migration of epithelial cells into the wound during healing

a. Allograft

b. Autologous graft

c. Bovine graft

d. Epithelialization

e. Implant

f. Porcine graft

g. Composite graft

h. Xenograft

MATCHING

Match each term with the correct definition.

19. _____ The incision is not closed; it is left open to heal from the bottom up

20. _____ The incision is left open and sutured at a later time

21. _____ The incision is sutured in layers at the end of the procedure

22. _____ A breakdown of the surgical incision during the healing period

23. _____ Abdominal contents spill out of the body through a ruptured or torn abdominal wall

24. _____ Bands of scar tissue between the body wall and viscera

25. _____ Excessive shrinkage of scar tissue that occurs during healing

26. _____ A narrow tract in tissue; the result of chronic infection

a. Evisceration

b. Adhesion

c. Third intention

d. Secondary intention

e. Dehiscence

f. Fistula

g. Primary intention

h. Contracture

Choose the best answer to complete the question or statement.

27. Suture materials are regulated by:
    a. FDA
    b. OSHA
    c. CDC
    d. ECRI

28. Composite suture is:
    a. Made of strands with two different sizes
    b. Twisted
    c. Non-absorbable
    d. Jacketed with another chemical

29. Suture sizes:
    a. Are determined by the type of material they are made from
    b. Vary with different materials
    c. Are the same across all materials
    d. None of the above

30. Suture breakage while being used by the surgeon is related to the:
    a. Tensile strength
    b. Presence of infection
    c. Patient's condition
    d. Suture material

31. Capillary action refers to a suture's:
    a. Use on capillaries
    b. Tendency to wick fluid
    c. Ability to resist breakage
    d. Color

32. This type of suture is never used in the urinary tract:
    a. Chromic
    b. Plain catgut
    c. Non-absorbable
    d. Polygycolic

33. This type of suture should be moistened before use:
    a. Polyglycolic
    b. Silk
    c. Polyester
    d. Chromic

34. Sutures are coated in order to:
    a. Make them visible in tissue
    b. Resist absorption
    c. Decrease wicking
    d. All of the above

35. Stainless steel sutures are somewhat difficult to handle because they:
    a. Are stiff
    b. Have sharp ends
    c. Can kink easily
    d. All of the above

36. The swage of a suture is:
    a. The degree of curvature of the needle
    b. The area where the suture is fixed to the needle
    c. The type of point
    d. The color

37. The reverse cutting needle:
    a. Contains a cutting edge on the outside edge
    b. Contains a cutting edge on the inside edge
    c. Does not prevent the suture from slicing through the tissue
    d. Is preferred for suturing fatty tissue

38. The double arm suture is used for:
    a. Closing the abdomen
    b. Closing the eyelid
    c. Closing lacerations of the liver
    d. Closing a round structure

39. A suture ligature is a suture-needle combination used to:
    a. Ligate tissue bundles containing blood vessels
    b. Ligate large vessels such as the femoral artery
    c. Ligate a capillary bed
    d. Tag a blood vessel

40. Sutures are passed to the surgeon:
    a. On a one-to-one basis
    b. Positioned so that they do not require repositioning
    c. As required
    d. All of the above

41. Eyed needles are threaded from the:
    a. Outside to the inside of the curvature
    b. Inside to the outside of the curvature

22 Minimally Invasive Endoscopic and Robotic-Assisted Surgery

Student's Name _____

FILL IN THE BLANKS

Fill in the blanks for these phrases and sentences about the imaging equipment used in minimally invasive surgery.

1. The _____ connects the light source to the camera head or telescope. It contains several thousand of

   _____ .

2. Before powering on or off the light source, it must be _____ .

3. Some models of camera heads do not require white _____ .

4. The camera control unit captures signals from the _____ and displays them on the _____ .

5. The _____ of the video system is the ratio of horizontal to vertical pixels.

6. To prevent the telescope lens from fogging the scrub may dip it in warm water or use a _____ .

7. One should always hold the telescope by its _____ .

8. The optical angle is the _____

   _____ .

9. Light cables should be stored _____ to keep them from breaking.

10. MIS instruments and telescopes must be checked each time they are prepared for sterilization. What specific checks must be made?

    a. _____

    b. _____

    c. _____

    d. _____

MULTIPLE CHOICE

Select the best answer.

11. In order to maximize visibility during laparoscopic MIS:
    a. The abdomen is inflated with carbon dioxide.
    b. The abdomen is inflated with nitrous oxide.
    c. Additional telescopes may be used.
    d. A Huston needle is used.

12. Continuous irrigation is used during MIS of the:
    a. Abdomen
    b. Joint capsule
    c. Muscle planes
    d. Ovaries

13. The _____ is used to remove tissue in small segments during MIS.
    a. Bridge
    b. Endocatch
    c. Specimen removal system
    d. Resectoscope

14. Direct capacitative coupling is:
    a. When an uninsulated monopolar instrument contacts an insulated instrument
    b. When electricity is transmitted to the tissue
    c. When electricity of one instrument is transmitted to another touching tissue
    d. A break in the insulation of an instrument causing loose current to escape

15. VATS is:
    a. Variegated anatomical transfer system
    b. Video anatomical transfer system
    c. Video ablative tumor surgery
    d. Video-assisted thoracic surgery

16. The control head contains the:
    a. Deflecting tip
    b. Control unit
    c. Optical system
    d. Insertion tube

17. All fiberoptic endoscopes must be _____ before reprocessing.
    a. Cleaned
    b. Sterilized
    c. Disinfected
    d. Cooled down

18. Cloudiness in the lens scope may mean _____ of the lens.
    a. Leakage
    b. Breakage
    c. Splitting
    d. Loosening

19. To increase the light of the camera image, you must increase the:
    a. White balance
    b. Cord power
    c. Gain
    d. Image intensifier

20. Robotic movement that moves left or right in space is called:
    a. Yaw
    b. Pitch
    c. Roll
    d. Reverse

21. Robotic movement that is up or down is called:
    a. Yaw
    b. Pitch
    c. Roll
    d. Reverse

22. Before robotic surgery begins, the robotic arms are placed in the correct location with respect to the central column. This is called:
    a. Sweet spot
    b. Alignment
    c. Arm relocation
    d. Docking

23. During robotic surgery, the surgeon has no:
    a. Direct contact with the tissues
    b. Haptic touch
    c. Sterile gown or gloves
    d. All of the above

24. One of the main roles of the scrub during robotic surgery is:
    a. Switching out the surgical instruments
    b. Suturing the tissues
    c. Managing the console
    d. Adjusting the patient's position

23 General Surgery

KEY TERMS

Differentiate between the terms.

1. Anastomosis vs. resection: _____

2. Sentinel node vs. lymph node: _____

3. Hook wire vs. aspiration needle: _____

4. Lobectomy vs. segmental resection: _____

5. Stoma vs. ostomy: _____

6. Billroth II vs. Billroth I: _____

7. Rectus sheath vs. linea alba: _____

8. Surgical mesh vs. Teflon sheet: _____

FILL IN THE BLANKS

Fill the blanks with the correct words to complete the sentences.

9. When performing resection of the stomach the **a.** _____ must be detached from the lesser and greater curvatures. When performing a resection of the bowel the **b.** _____ must be detached from the intestine in order to free up the sections. During mobilization of the gastrointestinal tract, energy devices are used these may include the **c.** _____ and **d.** _____. The small intestine can be accessed through the **e.** _____ cavity. The large intestine can be accessed through a **f.** _____ cavity and **g.** _____ cavity.

10. During procedures of the upper gastrointestinal tract, the operating table may be tipped into **a.** _____ _____ position in order to shift the abdominal viscera away from the target tissues. During lower pelvic procedures the operating table may be tipped into **b.** _____ position to shift the viscera away from the target tissues. When any change is made in the position of the operating table, the scrub may need to re-position the **c.** _____ to prevent it from coming in contact with the patient.

11. The Varess technique used to insufflate the abdomen requires a(n) **a.** _____ needle which is attached to the gas tubing. When using this the needle a **b.** _____ test is performed to ensure that the needle has not penetrated **c.** _____. In Hasson technique **d.** _____ are used to secure the trocar in place. The insufflation tubing is then attached to the _____.

12. The objective of using bowel technique is to prevent _____ _____.

13. The Roux-en-Y procedure results in an anastomosis between the **a.** _____ and

    b. _____. Another result is the anastomosis of the lower **c.** _____ to the upper

    d. _____. The Roux-en-Y is often performed for long term **e.** _____.

MATCHING

Match the words with their definition.

14. _____ Used to differentiate between nerves and blood vessels

15. _____ This is placed within a breast mass to identify the location

16. _____ Injected into a lymph chain to track probable cancerous tissues

17. _____ The entire breast is removed but the chest muscles are preserved

18. _____ The entire breast, all axillary nodes, and the chest wall muscles are removed

19. _____ This attaches the greater and lesser curvature of the stomach providing protection to the viscera

20. _____ This is used to protect and isolate the bowel during retroperitoneal procedures

21. _____ Used to retract large blood vessels

22. _____ Surgical technique used to free up structures from their surrounding support tissue

23. _____ Diagnostic endoscopy of the esophagus, stomach, and proximal duodenum

a. Radical mastectomy

b. Esophagogastroduodenostomy

c. Omentum

d. Hook (J) wire

e. Simple mastectomy

f. Vessel loop

g. Isofluran blue

h. Nerve stimulator

i. Bowel bag

j. Mobilization

24 Gynecological and Obstetrical Surgery

Student's Name _____

MULTIPLE CHOICE

Select the best answer to the question or phrase.

1. During gynecologic surgery the ureters must be identified and retracted gently. A _____ is often used to do this.
   a. Nerve root retractor
   b. Narrow Deaver
   c. Penrose drain
   d. U.S. retractor

2. Suction drains are placed at the close of radical surgery. An example of a suction drain is a _____.
   a. Mushroom drain
   b. Foley catheter
   c. Penrose drain
   d. Hemovac drain

3. Tissue morcellation is one technique used to remove a benign myoma. The _____ is commonly used in this technique.
   a. Resectoscope
   b. Tissue shaver
   c. Roller ball
   d. Vacuum ablator

4. During MIS gynecologic procedures, a _____ is placed in the cervix to change the position of the uterus.
   a. Inflatable cuff
   b. Blue ring
   c. Cervical dilator
   d. Uterine manipulator

5. Another name for leiomyoma is:
   a. Fibroid tumor
   b. Adnexa tumor
   c. Adenoma
   d. Myxomyoma

6. A missed abortion is:
   a. The products of conception have been expelled but the placenta retained
   b. Uterine bleeding without cervical dilation
   c. Undiagnosed and undetected embryonic or fetal demise (death)
   d. Suspected abortion

7. Draping materials for the removal of an ovarian cyst through a Pfannensteil incision will probably include:
   a. Transverse lap drape, incise drape, under buttocks pouch
   b. Stirrup drapes, four surgery towels, lithotomy drape
   c. Four towels, a half sheet, incise drape, transverse lap drape
   d. Transverse lap drape with perineal opening, perineal drape

8. Surgical management of an ectopic pregnancy may include the following options:
   a. Oophorotomy, hysterectomy, salpingectomy
   b. Salpingectomy, salpingostomy, removal of fetal remnants
   c. Hysterectomy, bilateral tubal ligation, removal of clots
   d. Oophorotomy, bilateral tubal ligation

9. A colpotomy ring is used to:
   a. Identify the cervix during total abdominal hysterectomy (TAH)
   b. Manipulate the cervix during TAH
   c. Maintain the position of the cervix
   d. Prevent the delivery of the uterus through the cervix

10. During tuboplasty, dye is instilled into the oviducts. This is done to:
    a. Identify the fallopian tube
    b. Detect a tumor of the fallopian tube
    c. Detect malignant areas of the fallopian tube
    d. Determine the patency of the fallopian tube

FILL IN THE BLANK

Provide the word that best fits in the sentences below regarding techniques in gynecologic surgery.

11. The uterus is supported on all sides by _____ tissue. During hysterectomy these structures must be divided to mobilize the uterus. Heavy _____ clamps are used to grasp the tissue in this part of the surgery. However, unlike the uterus, the fallopian tubes are _____. In order to prevent injury to the tubes, _____ clamps are used to manipulate them. During transcervical procedures the edge of the cervix is grasped with a _____. During childbirth the _____ is often incised to prevent deep tissues from tearing. Ablation of the uterine cavity is performed to treat _____. This procedure is often performed using a hysteroscope. In this procedure the uterine cavity is filled with _____. However, during a diagnostic D and C, the endometrial tissue is removed using _____. The tissue is collected on a _____.

MATCHING I

Match each term with the correct definition.

12. _____ Herniation of the bladder into the vaginal wall

13. _____ Mass that arises from the germ layers of the embryo; may contain tissue remnants, including hair and teeth

14. _____ Endometrial tissue that implants outside of the uterine cavity

15. _____ Fibrous, benign tumor of the uterus that usually arises from the myometrium

16. _____ Caused by stretching and weakness of the uterine ligaments

17. _____ Infection which causes scarring of the fallopian tubes and adhesions in the abdominal and pelvic cavity often associated with infertility

18. _____ Bulging of intestinal tissue into a weakened posterior vaginal wall

19. _____ Excessive menstrual bleeding

20. _____ Diagnosed in women with persistent multiple cystic follicles

21. _____ Implantation of the embryo outside the uterus

22. _____ A follicle that does not regress after releasing an egg

a. Ovarian cyst

b. Dermoid cyst

c. Polycystic ovary syndrome

d. Uterine prolapse

e. Cystocele

f. Pelvic inflammatory disease (PID)

g. Rectocele

h. Ectopic pregnancy

i. Leiomyoma

j. Menorrhagia

k. Endometriosis

MATCHING II

Match the surgical procedure with the correct definition. You may use the same answer more than once.

24. _____ Removal of a circumferential core of tissue around the cervix

25. _____ Female sterilization procedure

26. _____ The removal of the uterus by a combined laparoscopic and vaginal approach

27. _____ The uterus is surgically removed through a pelvic incision

28. _____ Surgical removal of the uterus and cervix

29. _____ Surgical removal of the ovaries, fallopian tubes, supporting ligaments, upper vagina, and pelvic lymph nodes

30. _____ A fiberoptic hysteroscope is inserted through the cervix and into the uterus

31. _____ Removal of a benign leiomyoma of the myometrium to control bleeding and prevent pressure on other structures in the pelvis

32. _____ Sharp and smooth curettes are used to remove the surface of the endometrium through a transvaginal approach

33. _____ Herniated tissue of the anterior and posterior vagina is reduced, and the vaginal walls are reconstructed

34. _____ A sinus tract between the rectum and the vagina

a. LAVH

b. Total abdominal hysterectomy

c. Laparoscopic tubal ligation

d. Anterior-posterior repair

e. Hysteroscopy

f. Cone biopsy of the cervix

g. Vesicovaginal fistula

h. Radical hysterectomy

i. Myomectomy

j. Dilation and curettage

k. Vaginal hysterectomy

CASE STUDY

A 59-year-old patient has been diagnosed with endometrial cancer and admitted for a radical hysterectomy with bilateral lymphadenectomy. The procedure will be performed through a midline incision and is expected to take 3 hours.

1. What anatomical structures will be sent for pathology?

2. What specific patient care is required between the time the patient is transported to the OR and the patient is anesthetized?

111

3. Which abdominal self-retaining retractors might be used in this procedure?

4. What size and type of suture might be used on the uterine ligaments?

5. How will the lymph nodes be managed on the back table? How will they be identified and labeled?

6. Will the retroperitoneum be entered in this procedure?

7. What instrument sets will be required for the procedure?

8. Will a vaginal prep be necessary for the procedure? Provide the rationale in your answer.

25 Genitourinary Surgery

Student's Name _____

FILL IN THE BLANKS

Fill in the word that best fits these statements about endoscopic and minimally invasive equipment.

1. The a. _____ is a round-tip rod inserted into the sheath to prevent injury to the b. _____ during insertion of the cystourethroscope. The Albarran is a type of c. _____. This connects the d. _____ to the telescope. The e. _____ cystourethroscope requires a fiberoptic light source and cable. Routine cystoscopy is performed with the flexible or f. _____ cystourethroscope. A 0° telescope sees g. _____, while a 30° scope view is h. _____. Either i. _____ or j. _____ can be used for continuous irrigation during routine *diagnostic* cystoscope.

MULTIPLE CHOICE

Select the best answer to the question.

2. During transurethral resection of the bladder a tumor is commonly removed using a resectoscope and

   _____.
   a. Cutting loop
   b. Bipolar electrode
   c. Roller ball
   d. Flexible cystoscope

3. Implantation of radioactive seeds in the cancerous prostate is called:
   a. Gamma therapy
   b. Radioactive chemotherapy
   c. Brachytherapy
   d. Trachotherapy

4. In percutaneous nephrolithotomy, a nephroscope is passed through the:
   a. Urethra, ureter, and renal pelvis
   b. Tissues of the back into the kidney
   c. Space of Retzius and into the kidney
   d. Iliac fossa and into the kidney

5. Following nephrolithotomy, what type of drain is placed in the kidney pelvis?
   a. Hemovac or Jackson Pratt
   b. Malecot or Pezzer
   c. Stainless steel stent
   d. J loop

SHORT ANSWER

Answer the question using *one or more* short answers.

6. Select the instruments that are appropriate to mobilize the ureter from its connective tissue attachments.

   a. DeBakey vascular forceps

   b. Mayo scissors (curved)

   c. Pean clamps

   d. Metzenbaum scissors

   e. Sponge dissector

f. Allis clamp

   g. Kidney pedicle clamp

   h. Right angle clamp

7. Kidney transplant requires which instrument sets and extras (recipient only)?

   a. Plastic surgery

   b. Major kidney set

   c. Vascular set

   d. General surgery

   e. Gastrointestinal set

   f. Right angle clamps

   g. Ultrasonic shears

   h. Vascular sutures

8. The Foley catheter can be used for these purposes:

   a. Intermittent bladder drainage

   b. As a tamponade

   c. Bladder irrigation

   d. Continuous bladder drainage

   e. To instill medication

   f. To decompress the stomach before surgery

   g. As a stent following ureteral surgery

9. A ureteral stent can be used to:

   a. Support the ureter

   b. Drain the kidney

   c. Drain the bladder

   d. Illuminate the ureter

   e. Bypass a stone

   f. Retrieve a stone

   g. Insert a guidewire

CRITICAL THINKING EXERCISE

As a student you learned the basic concepts of genitourinary surgery, including endoscopic techniques. However, in your new job you have been asked to step in for the cysto technician who will be absent from work for 3 days. The first day was very difficult, but the urologist was helpful. On the second day you began to understand why certain techniques are used. On the third day you were much more confident assisting. However, there is still a lot you are not familiar with, especially the location and types of equipment used in your facility. Now you realize that a cysto manual needs to be written to help other technologists who are new to this specialty area.

Make an outline of topics you think should be covered in a basic orientation manual for your particular cysto room. For example, one topic might be "Types of stents in stock." You only need to list the topics, not the techniques or details about procedures.

26 Ophthalmic Surgery

Student's Name _____

Fill in the blanks.

1. The anterior chamber is filled with a liquid called a. _____. This chamber lies in front of the b. _____. The posterior chamber lies in front of the c. _____ and behind the d. _____. Fluid passes from the anterior to posterior chamber through the e. _____. This fluid exits the eye through the f. _____, and passes into the g. _____.

2. The eye prep is performed using a. _____% b. _____. The prep starts at the c. _____. Sponges that touch the d. _____ during the prep must be discarded, as this area is contaminated. During draping it is important to isolate the e. _____.

3. All sponges used in eye surgery must be a. _____ to prevent particles from entering the eye. The scrub is required to sponge the eye during surgery. This is done by b. _____ _____. It is important never to touch the c. _____ with a sponge.

4. The a. _____ is the lighting system of the microscope. The b. _____ provides the greatest magnification. The c. _____ increases and decreases magnification. When moving the microscope it is necessary to first d. _____. It must also be balanced. This is necessary in order to e. _____. When moving the microscope, always grasp it by the f. _____ to prevent it from tipping.

LABELING

5. Label the following parts of the lacrimal system.

1. _____

2. _____

3. _____

4. _____

5. _____

6. _____

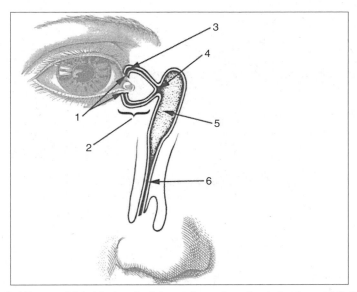

From Albert D, Miller J, *Albert and Jakobiec's principles and practice of opthalmology*, ed 3, Philadelphia, 2008, Saunders

MULTIPLE CHOICE

Select the best answer to complete the sentence.

6. During dacryocystorhinostomy, small bone ronguers are needed to:
   a. Open the sphenoid bone
   b. Make an opening in the nasal bone
   c. Enlarge the opening in the lacrimal bone
   d. Perform an osteotomy in the orbital ridge

7. During strabismus surgery, this instrument is used to elevate and mobilize the muscle.
   a. Stevens muscle hook
   b. Chalazion clamp
   c. Mosquito clamp
   d. Bridle suture

8. A trephine is used in corneal transplant to:
   a. Incise the iris
   b. Harvest a graft
   c. Guide the placement of sutures
   d. Produce a button of tissue

9. The phrase "open sky" refers to a condition resulting from:
   a. Exposure of the pupil to light
   b. Exposure of the iris to light
   c. Removal of the cornea
   d. Loss of vitreous

10. The significance of open sky is:
    a. It exposes the optic nerve to contamination.
    b. It exposes the anterior chamber to the environment.
    c. It may result in loss of vitreous humor.
    d. It exposes the posterior chamber to contamination.

11. Phacoemulsification is the preferred method of cataract removal for most patients because:
    a. Only the target tissue is removed.
    b. The zonules can be safety removed.
    c. The lens capsule can extracted.
    d. The lens capsule is liquefied.

117

12. Retinal detachment occurs when the retina is torn and is extended by:
    a. The loss of vitreous from the posterior chamber to the anterior chamber
    b. The aging process
    c. Vitreous seeping between the pigment layer and neural layer
    d. Vitreous leakage into the globe causing the eye to collapse

13. A scleral buckle is a:
    a. Silastic sponge and band encircling the sclera
    b. Cable tie type of band placed around the Tenon capsule
    c. Stainless steel buckle sutured to the Tenon capsule
    d. Metal strip encircling the sclera

14. The purpose of the bridle suture is:
    a. To fix the globe in one position during surgery
    b. To rotate the globe during surgery
    c. To provide flexibility to the sclera
    d. To prevent the loss of vitreous from the eye

15. During enucleation, a sphere is placed in the orbital cavity. This is done to:
    a. Maintain the shape of the cavity
    b. Prevent infection
    c. Prevent the optic nerve from prolapsing
    d. Push the remaining tissues posteriorly

CASE STUDY

1. What are the suspected causes of toxic anterior segment syndrome (TASS)?

2. What steps should be taken at the close of cataract surgery to prevent TASS?

27 Surgery of the Ear, Nose, Pharynx, and Larynx

Student's Name _____

MULTIPLE CHOICE

Select the best answer to complete the sentence.

1. Hemostasis during ear surgery is maintained using:
   a. Suture ligatures
   b. Gelfoam and epinephrine
   c. Balance saline solution (BSS)
   d. Cold saline solution

2. The middle ear contains the three bones of sound transmission; these are the:
   a. Ossicle, stapes, hammer
   b. Hammer, stapes, uncus
   c. Incus, stapes, malleus
   d. Hammer, incus, organ of Corti

3. The skin prep for ear surgery may include:
   a. The periauicular area
   b. The middle ear
   c. The ossicles
   d. The shoulder

4. A non-healing hole in the tympanic membrane may be repaired using a:
   a. Myringotomy tube
   b. Gelatine sponge
   c. Fat graft
   d. Silastic patch

5. Mastoidectomy literally means:
   a. Removal of mastoid bone
   b. Removal of a cholesteatoma
   c. Removal of a tumor
   d. Removal of the organ of Corti

6. One of the last steps in a mastoidectomy is to pack the mastoid cavity and middle ear with:
   a. Bone wax
   b. Methylmethacrylate
   c. Iodophor gauze
   d. Gelfoam

7. The most common indication for a stapedectomy is:
   a. Osteoporosis
   b. Osteomalacia
   c. Osteosclerosis
   d. Cholesteatoma

MATCHING I

Match each term with the correct definition.

8. _____ A benign tumor of the middle ear caused by shedding of keratin in chronic otitis media

9. _____ Defect that can be caused by a blast injury or penetrating foreign body in the ear

10. _____ Enlargement of an organ or anatomical structure

11. _____ Transmits sounds directly to the 8th cranial nerve

12. _____ Fluid in the middle ear

13. _____ Bleeding arising from the nasal cavity

14. _____ Vibration of the vocal cords during speaking or vocalization

15. _____ Paralysis of a structure

16. _____ Excessive proliferation of mucosal epithelium

17. _____ Hearing impairment arising from the cochlea, auditory nerve, or central nervous system

a. Cholesteatoma

b. Phonation

c. Polyp

d. Perforation of the TM

e. Epistaxis

f. Effusion

g. Hypertrophy

h. Sensorineural hearing loss

i. Cochlear implant

j. Paresis

FILL IN THE BLANK

Provide a term that completes the sentence.

18. During tonsillectomy, it is common practice to hold the mouth in an open position using a _____ that is attached to the _____ .

19. During adenoidectomy, the _____ must be retracted superiorly. This is frequently done using a _____ .

20. The patient skin prep is omitted for procedures of the mouth because _____ .

21. Before inserting the rigid laryngoscope, a _____ must be placed in the mouth.

22. After tracheostomy, the obturator must be kept with the patient at all times. The obturator is used to _____ .

23. The narrow band of tissue separating the thyroid lobes is called the _____ .

24. During thyroidectomy, the scrub should have many _____ available because the gland is highly vascular.

25. The SCM referred to in procedures of the neck is the _____ .

26. A power saw and drill should be available for a glossectomy because _____ .

CRITICAL THINKING EXERCISE

Facial nerve paralysis is a devastating complication of head and neck surgery.

1. What supplies or equipment is used to *retract* a major nerve?

2. Which device is used to aid in *identification* of the facial nerve?

3. Name the instruments that might be used to mobilize the facial nerve.

Student's Name _____

IDENTIFICATION

Study the illustration below and list the following:

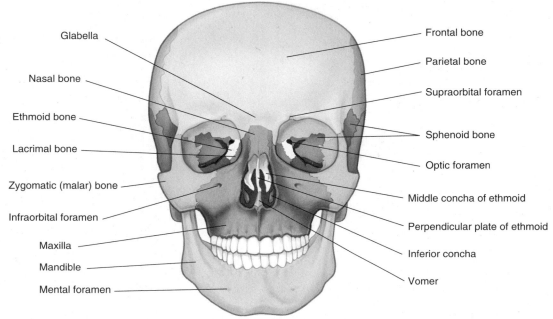

Glabella

Nasal bone

Ethmoid bone

Lacrimal bone

Zygomatic (malar) bone

Infraorbital foramen

Maxilla

Mandible

Mental foramen

Frontal bone

Parietal bone

Supraorbital foramen

Sphenoid bone

Optic foramen

Middle concha of ethmoid

Perpendicular plate of ethmoid

Inferior concha

Vomer

From Thibodeau GA, Patt KT: *Anthony's textbook of anatomy and physiology*, ed 17, St Louis, 2003, Mosby.

1. Bones of the midface

_____

_____

_____

2. Bones of the upper face

_____

_____

_____

3. Bones of the lower face

_____

_____

_____

MULTIPLE CHOICE

Select the best answer to complete the sentence.

4. The primary means of repairing a facial fracture is:
   a. Fibrin glue and nails
   b. Arch bars
   c. Plates and screws
   d. Silicone implants

5. A resorbable implant is:
   a. One that is slowly absorbed by the body
   b. A biomechanical system made of titanium
   c. Made of a combination of silicone and Teflon
   d. Heated to 212° before implantation

6. A serious risk in facial fracture is:
   a. Damage to the nasal bone
   b. Maintaining the airway
   c. Inability to open the mouth
   d. Leakage of CSF

7. A blowout fracture may result in:
   a. Extrusion of the eye into the nasal sinus
   b. Entrapment of the eye muscles
   c. Displacement of the globe posteriorly
   d. All of the above

8. The application of arch bars is:
   a. Wiring the orbital rim to the maxillary sinus
   b. Wiring the teeth to the zygoma
   c. Wiring the hard palate to the maxilla
   d. Wiring the mandible to the maxilla

9. Arch bars may:
   a. Be removed at the end of the surgical procedure
   b. Interfere with normal respiration
   c. Be left in place for 3 to 6 months
   d. Be left in place until the orbital rim heals

10. Before repairing fractures of the face, it is important to:
    a. Assess the patient for blood borne disease
    b. Assess the patient for other injuries
    c. Identify the witnesses to the incident that caused the fractures
    d. Obtain x-rays from the patient's dentist

11. Facial fractures should be repaired as soon as possible because:
    a. The patient will develop uncontrollable hemorrhage
    b. The soft tissues will swell
    c. The patient is in severe pain
    d. The patient might develop an infection

12. When preparing the plates or metal mesh to repair a fracture, the scrub should have:
    a. Several lengths of arch bar material
    b. Metzenbaum scissors
    c. A cartilage press
    d. A plate bender and pliers

13. If a drill guide is used to stabilize the drill bit when making screw holes:
    a. A plate holding forceps and depth gauge may be needed
    b. The length of the screw is predetermined
    c. Only a magnetic drill guide should be used
    d. The drill guide is pre-set for the length of the screw

Study the illustration below.

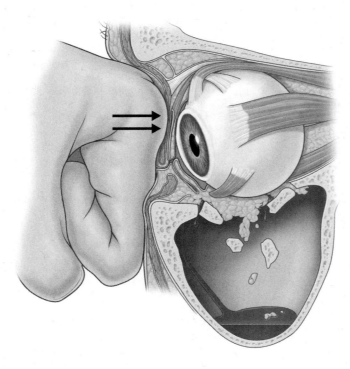

From Neligan P, Buck D, *Core procedures in plastic surgery*, 2014, Elsevier

1. Based on what you have learned in this and other chapters, describe what instrument sets you should have for surgical management of the trauma. You may also include special instruments, supplies, and devices.

   Bonus points: Can you name the structure where blood is seen collecting from the trauma?

29 Plastic and Reconstructive Surgery

Student's Name _____

MULTIPLE CHOICE

Select the best answer to complete the sentence.

1. The skin layer that contains blood vessels and nerves is the:
   a. Stratum germinativum
   b. Stratum lucidum
   c. Dermis
   d. Epidermis

2. The SMAS includes the tissue layers of the face. SMAS stands for:
   a. Subcutaneous muscle and stratum
   b. Superficial musculoaponeurotic system
   c. Subcutaneous musculoappendicular system
   d. Superficial musculoappendicular stratum

3. A full thickness skin graft is composed of:
   a. Epidermis, dermis, fatty tissue
   b. Epidermis, dermis
   c. Epidermis, fatty tissue, muscle
   d. None of the above

4. A split thickness skin graft contains:
   a. Dermis only
   b. Epidermis only
   c. Stratum lucidum only
   d. Stratus corneum only

5. Common donor sites for a split thickness graft include the:
   a. Buttock, lateral thigh, back, abdomen
   b. Inguinal crease, back, lower leg, forearm
   c. Buttock, lateral thigh, lower leg, forearm
   d. Buttock, back, upper arm, inguinal crease

6. Common donor sites for a full thickness graft include the:
   a. Decubital space, inguinal crease, lateral thigh
   b. Lower abdomen, inguinal crease, upper thigh
   c. Buttock fold, infrabdominal fold, anterior wrist, elbow fold
   d. Lower abdomen, lateral thigh, buttock, neck

7. A skin graft mesher is used to:
   a. Score the skin before a graft is taken
   b. Flatten a skin graft for better adherence
   c. Stretch the skin while the graft is being taken
   d. Cut holes in the graft to allow fluid to escape during healing

8. A xenograft is one that is:
   a. Harvested from one animal species and placed in another species
   b. Harvested from the patient and placed in another location
   c. Harvested from one person for use in another person
   d. None of the above

9. A bovine graft comes from:
   a. Pig tissue
   b. A synthetic absorbable polymer
   c. Tissue of a cow
   d. Tissue from another person

10. Mohs surgery is a method used to:
    a. Map out a tumor
    b. Identify the boundaries of a tumor
    c. Determine the margins of a tumor
    d. All of the above

11. When passing the dermatome to the surgeon, the ST must first:
    a. Disassemble it
    b. Assemble it and set the blade on zero
    c. Apply mineral oil to the blade
    d. Pull the donor site taut using a tongue blade

12. A carrier plate is used to:
    a. Release the graft from the dermatome
    b. Carry the graft from the donor site to the back table
    c. Hold the graft during meshing
    d. Hold the graft while the surgeon trims it

13. A pedicle graft is used to:
    a. Prevent infection at the recipient site
    b. Transfer skin cells to the recipient site
    c. Extend the recipient site
    d. Provide vascularizatioin to the recipient site

14. A pedicle graft may also be called a:
    a. Flap graft
    b. Free graft
    c. Near graft
    d. Distant graft

MATCHING

Select the word that applies.

15. _____ Absorbed by the body but not derived from biological tissue

16. _____ Derived from living tissue

17. _____ Zig-zag incision

18. _____ Tissue is smooth and shiny with dry blisters and edema

19. _____ Chin implant surgery

20. _____ Tissue may be white, brown, or black; appears waxy

21. _____ Breast attachment tissue is pulled superiorly

22. _____ Charred tissue

a. Third-degree burn

b. Eschar

c. Mastopexy

d. Second-degree burn

e. Biosynthetic

f. Mentoplasty

g. Biological graft

h. Z-plasty

FILL IN THE BLANK

Fill in the blanks with the appropriate words.

23. A TRAM flap is a type of _____ graft.

   "TRAM" means _____ .

24. In a TRAM procedure tissue is brought from the _____ to the

   _____ site through a tunnel in the _____ .

25. The DIEP technique is an alternative to the TRAM flap. In this technique _____ instruments
   are required in addition to general surgery and breast instruments.

INTEGRATION OF KNOWLEDGE

Match the instrument with the set in which it belongs. You may select more than one instruments per set.

26. _____ Carrier plate

27. _____ Ballenger swivel knife

28. _____ Aufrict retractor

29. _____ Wire cutters

30. _____ Fiberoptic retractor

31. _____ Short tenotomy scissors

32. _____ Deaver retractor

33. _____ Bone clamp

34. _____ Dermatome

35. _____ Button knife

36. _____ Extractor

37. _____ Screws

38. _____ Plate bender

a. Basic plastic surgery

b. Rhinoplasty

c. Breast surgery

d. Maxillofacial

e. Oral

f. Skin graft

g. Rhytidectomy

30 Orthopedic Surgery

Student's Name _____

FILL IN THE BLANK

Fill in the blank with a word that completes the sentence.

1. Bone, ligaments, and tendons are all types of _____ tissue.

2. A ligament connects _____ to bone. A tendon connects _____ to

   _____.

3. A flat sheet of fascia to which muscles attach is called a(n) _____.

4. The tough fibrous tissue covering long bones is called _____.

5. Joints that have a capsule are filled with an oily substance called _____ _____.

6. It is important to understand the normal range of motion of a joint to prevent _____ to the patient during moving and handling.

MULTIPLE CHOICE

Select the best word or phrase to answer the questions.

7. A topical hemostatic substance used on bone is called:
   a. Surgicel
   b. Ostene
   c. Gelfoam
   d. Avitene

8. Infection control in orthopedic surgery is critical because:
   a. Most fractures are contaminated.
   b. There are many people in the operating room, which increases the risk of infection.
   c. Postoperative infection in bone may result in long-term or chronic disability.
   d. Postoperative infection in the bone may require antibiotics.

9. Orthopedic injuries are treated as soon as possible after the trauma occurs because:
   a. There is usually severe bleeding.
   b. Most accidents occur at night.
   c. The patient can become septic.
   d. Severe tissue swelling occurring hours after the trauma makes the procedure more difficult.

10. When a fracture is scheduled, it is important for the scrub to know what type it is because:
    a. The insurance company may question team members.
    b. He or she needs to know how long the surgery will take.
    c. Case planning depends on it.
    d. The on-call team may need to be called.

11. Bleeding a power instrument refers to:
    a. Draining the gas from the hose while the instrument is in the off position
    b. Draining the gas from the hose before handing the instrument to the surgeon
    c. Placing the instrument on "safety" before handing it to the surgeon
    d. Draining all lubricant from the head before sterilization

MATCHING

Match the surgery with its classifications. Use two answers for each fraction—one for reduction and one for fixation.

12. _____ An incision is made in the leg and a metal plate, and screws are used to bridge the fracture.

13. _____ The broken bones are aligned using manual traction and a cast is applied with the patient under deep sedation.

14. _____ The patient is given a general anesthetic, and the fractured bone is pulled into alignment. Fixation pins are drilled through the skin and into the bone. These are connected with a metal frame.

15. _____ An incision is made over the fractured femur. The bone ends are drawn into alignment using bone clamps. A nail is inserted to hold the bone fragments together. The incision is closed.

16. _____ A fractured arm is x-rayed showing the bone fragments in alignment. A cast is applied.

17. _____ A comminuted open fracture of the leg is repaired through the existing trauma wound using multiple plates and pins. The wound is closed. A soft stabilizing dressing and brace are applied.

a. Open reduction

b. Closed reduction

c. Open fixation

d. Closed fixation

MATCHING

Match the implant terminology with its description.

18. _____ Used with threaded screw holes

19. _____ Makes a hole as it is drilled

20. _____ Contains locking screws

21. _____ Intramedullary nail

22. _____ Has a hollow core

23. _____ Thick sharp wire drilled into bone fragments

24. _____ Pulls the bone fragments together as it is fixed using compression

25. _____ A threaded plug with heavy cord attached to fix ligaments and tendon to bone

26. _____ A type of joint implant that requires no cement; it is impacted into the bone

27. _____ Melded using plate benders to fit the bone

a. Anchor screw

b. Self-tapping

c. Locking screw

d. Press fit

e. Lag screw

f. Impacted into the medullary canal of both bone fragments to hold them in alignment

g. Reconstruction plate

h. Cannulated

i. Kirchsner wire

j. Locking plate

FILL IN THE BLANK

Fill in the blanks to complete the sentences.

28. Recurrent dislocation of the glenohumeral joint is often caused when the a. _____ becomes torn. This causes the glenoid capsule to become shallow, and the b. _____ is forced out of the joint. Surgery is performed to reattach the c. _____ to the glenoid rim.

29. Rotator cuff repair involves attaching the a. _____ of the rotator cuff to the b. _____. This can be accomplished with sutures or c. _____. Sometimes an acromioplasty is performed in the same procedure. This involves removing any d. _____ on the anterior acromion.

30. During arthroplasty one or both components of the shoulder joint are replaced with a. _____. Replacement of the humerus requires reaming of the medullary canal. This is performed using b. _____. The most common entry incision for shoulder arthroplasty is the c. _____. The humeral head is severed using a(n) d. _____.

31. The most common wrist injury is fracture of the a. _____ bone. Usually a cannulated b. _____ is used to bridge the bone fragments. An example is the c. _____.

32. During hip fracture surgery, the orthopedic table is often used. In this technique, the operative leg is placed in a boot in order to apply a. _____. The femoral neck or b. _____ is a common site of fracture. A common method of repair is to fix a c. _____ screw through the bone fragments with a d. _____ attached to the femur. In this procedure a e. _____ pin is required to establish the correct angle for the screw. To install the side plate, a drill, f. _____, and g. _____ are required.

33. During hip arthroplasty modular implants may be used. These are the a. _____ component and the b. _____ component. A(n) c. _____ must be performed to remove the femoral head. When cleaning the acetabulum the surgeon may use d. _____ and a power e. _____. Just as in shoulder arthroplasty, f. _____ are used to open the medullary canal.

34. Fracture of the pelvis can be life threatening because a. _____ _____. A b. _____ may be applied to the pelvis by EMTs in the field in order to c. _____. A d. _____ incision is commonly used to expose the fractures. The fractures are commonly reduced using e. _____. Fixation usually requires f. _____ held in place by g. _____.

35. Knee arthroscopy is commonly used for repair of soft tissue injury. During the procedure the knee joint is a. _____ using b. _____ solution. Repair of the ACL may require a c. _____ taken from the patellar tendon.

36. A tibial fracture is often repaired using an intramedullary rod or nail placed in the a. _____ of the tibia. During the procedure b. _____ are used to verify the position of instruments and the implant. Once the pin is in place, c. _____ _____ are used to prevent the pin from rotating.

37. Amputation of a limb is classified as a. _____ or b. _____. These refer to the blood supply to the limb. Skin flaps are created, and myodesis is performed to fix the c. _____ to the d. _____. However this technique is only applied to a(n) e. _____.

CASE STUDY

1. Your patient is undergoing a hip replacement and will be placed in lateral position with both arms extended on armboards. List the positioning accessories needed, where they are placed, and why.

31 Peripheral Vascular Surgery

Student's Name _____

MATCHING

Match the procedure with its definition.

1. _____ Removal of a blood clot, atherosclerotic material, or other obstruction from an artery

2. _____ An endovascular minimally invasive procedure to repair a blood vessel

3. _____ Removal of a blood clot from a major artery

4. _____ An incision made in an artery

5. _____ Method used to introduce and exchange consecutive guidewires and stents into a vessel by fitting one over the other

6. _____ A method of registering and measuring blood flow using ultrasound

7. _____ Minimally invasive procedure to repair an aortic aneurysm

8. _____ A surgical procedure to establish a new path of circulation using an existing blood vessel

9. _____ Anastomosis of a vein and artery for dialysis access

10. _____ Establishing a path of blood flow using a graft

a. Endarterectomy

b. Seldinger technique

c. EVAR

d. Doppler scanning

e. Thrombectomy

f. Percutaneous angioplasty

g. Arteriotomy

h. Creation of an arteriovenous shunt

i. Bypass grafting

j. In situ bypass

MULTIPLE CHOICE

Select the best answer.

11. This drug is used in solution to irrigate blood vessels during anastomosis.
    a. Saline for irrigation
    b. Topical thrombin
    c. 25% Vispaque
    d. Heparinized saline

12. This drug stimulates the body's clotting mechanism.
    a. Thrombin
    b. Low molecular weight heparin
    c. BSS
    d. Liquid collagen

13. Must be used for reconstitution of human or bovine thrombin.
    a. 0.9% sodium chloride for irrigation
    b. Sterile water
    c. 0.9% sodium chloride intravenous
    d. 1% xylocaine intravenous

14. This drug is supplied in powder form for use on bleeding anastomosis sites.
    a. Collagen
    b. Fibrinogen
    c. PFTE
    d. Methylmethacrylate

15. This drug causes vasodilation and is used when a vein is harvested for an autograft.
    a. Carbachol
    b. Atropine
    c. Oxytocin
    d. Papaverine

16. This type of catheter is used to enlarge the lumen of a vessel.
    a. Exchange catheter
    b. Guidewire
    c. Angioplasty balloon catheter
    d. Sizing catheter

17. This device is used as a pilot for the insertion of other devices in the artery.
    a. Guidewire
    b. Stent
    c. Balloon catheter
    d. Measuring catheter

18. This type of device is used to wall off sclerotic plaque and keep the vessel open.
    a. Guidewire
    b. Stent
    c. Angiocatheter
    d. Angioplasty balloon

19. When inflating an angioplasty balloon, an insufflation device is used to:
    a. Inflate the balloon to the correct pressure
    b. Inject contrast dye into the blood vessel
    c. Expand the blood vessel during angiography
    d. Inject air into the artery

20. During endarterectomy, which instrument can be used to dissect plaque from the vessel wall?
    a. Rosen pick
    b. Sclerotomy knife
    c. Penfield elevator
    d. Freer curette

FILL IN THE BLANK

Fill in the blank with the correct word.

21. A dissecting aneurysm is one in which the _____

    _____ .

22. During aneurysm repair a _____ graft may be used to bypass the aneurysm.

23. The prep area for an abdominal aneurysm extends from the a. _____to the b. _____

    _____ .

24. When the retroperitoneum is entered, a _____ may be needed to contain the viscera.

25. A common type forceps used in vascular surgery are the _____

    _____ .

26. In aortofemoral bypass, the _____ is (are) bypassed to restore circulation.

27. The surgical term *shunt* means _____ .

28. Two devices used in vascular surgery to monitor blood flow are the _____
    and the _____

    _____ .

29. Varicose vein stripping is performed to treat _____

    _____ .

30. Following percutaneous procedures of the femoral artery, a _____

    _____ dressing is necessary.

Mr. X has been admitted for a left carotid endarterectomy. Based on what you have learned about this procedure, write up a Surgeon's Preference Card as it might appear for this procedure. It is not necessary to list standard items such as drapes, gowns, gloves, ESU, and so on. You may need to consult other chapters. Be sure to include the following information:

a. Patient position

b. Skin prep instructions

c. Instrument sets needed

d. "Special instruments needed"

e. Sponges and accessory items (e.g., clamp shods)

f. Drugs and solutions needed

g. Medical devices

h. Dressings

Thoracic and Pulmonary Surgery

Student's Name _____

MATCHING

Match the procedure with its definition.

1. _____ An outpatient procedure in which ultrasound guidance is used to stage lymph nodes

2. _____ Removal of thrombus in a pulmonary vessel

3. _____ Minimally invasive surgery to map and biopsy tumors in the peripheral tissues of the lung

4. _____ Removal of the entire lung

5. _____ Portions of the lung affected by pulmonary emphysema are removed

6. _____ A specific lobe of the lung is removed

7. _____ Surgical treatment for empyema

8. _____ Minimally invasive thoracic surgery performed through ports in the chest wall

9. _____ Endoscopic surgery of the mediastinal space

a. Electromagnetic navigation bronchoscopy

b. Pneumonectomy

c. Lung volume reduction

d. Pulmonary thromboembolectomy

e. Endobronchial ultrasound

f. Mediastinoscopy

g. VATS

h. Lobectomy

i. Decortication

MULTIPLE CHOICE

Select the best answer.

10. An underwater closed chest seal drainage system is needed to:
    a. Restore positive pressure in the pleural space
    b. Remove exudate from the mediastinum
    c. Restore negative pressure in the pleural space
    d. All of the above

11. If the underwater chest drainage system is positioned higher than the chest:
    a. Fluid can fill the pleural space, preventing ventilation
    b. Fluid can spill out of the system and create a health hazard
    c. Air may enter the system, causing positive pressure in the pleural space
    d. The system may overflow, causing negative pressure in the pleural space

12. During an open thoracotomy through a posterolateral incision, it is necessary to:
    a. Place a magnetic instrument pad near the surgical wound
    b. Wrap the ESU cord around a hemostat to keep it from dropping off the field
    c. Place the suction near the head of the patient
    d. Place a needle pad near the incision

13. During a thoracotomy, a rib may be removed using:
    a. A rib approximator
    b. A Kerrison rongeur
    c. Bethune shears
    d. A rib rasp

14. A common self-retaining retractor used in thoracotomy is the:
    a. O'Sullivan O'Connor
    b. Finochietto
    c. Balfour
    d. Gelpi

15. Atraumatic clamps that may be used in thoracic surgery include the:
    a. Pean, Bainbridge, Payr
    b. Herrick, Babcock
    c. Bulldog, Glover
    d. Duval, Foerester

16. Surgical stapling instruments are commonly used in thoracic surgery to:
    a. Resect a lung
    b. Close the bronchus
    c. Obtain a tissue specimen
    d. All of the above

17. This product is used to seal a bronchial anastomosis.
    a. Gelfoam
    b. Ostene
    c. Epinephrine
    d. Fibrin

18. The rigid bronchoscope is required for:
    a. Diagnostic procedures
    b. Procedures requiring a wide bore
    c. Brush biopsy
    d. Procedures which use suction and irrigation

19. When sputum or fluid samples are required, a _____ is attached to the suction tubing.
    a. Mesh bag
    b. Likas tube
    c. Mican trap
    d. Lukens trap

FILL IN THE BLANK

Fill in the blanks to finish the sentences.

20. _____ refers to a bluish tint seen in patients with poor oxygenation.

21. Emphysema results in constriction of the _____.

22. Pneumothorax refers to _____.

23. Hemothorax refers to _____.

24. The lungs are separated in the thoracic cavity by the _____.

25. Cytology specimens are taken during bronchoscopy using a _____.

26. During endobronchial ultrasound, lymph nodes are identified for pathology according to their _____.

27. During VATS trocar sizes, _____ and _____ are commonly used.

28. Hemostasis can be maintained on a severed rib using _____.

29. The trachea is composed mainly of _____ tissue.

CASE STUDY

Provide a list of 10 instruments used specifically in a thoracotomy. Focus on instruments that are specific to thoracic surgery rather than general surgery. Include surgical stapling devices. Instruments of any category can be included (e.g., grasping, holding, occluding, and viewing). Describe what each instrument is specifically used for.

33 Cardiac Surgery

MATCHING

Select the procedure that fits the description.

1. ___ Implantation of this device is performed when a patient cannot be taken off CPB

2. ___ Surgery to correct a hole in the interatrial septum

3. ___ Harvested for use during CABG

4. ___ Performed to correct valve stenosis

5. ___ Open procedure performed to correct cardiac arrhythmias caused by a disease of the conduction system

6. ___ The most commonly used incision for cardiac surgery

7. ___ Performed to restore circulation to the heart muscle

8. ___ The inframammary internal mammary artery is an autograft for this procedure

9. ___ Performed as an alternative to mitral valve replacement

a. MIDCAB

b. Median sternotomy

c. Mitral commissurotomy

d. CABG

e. Intra-aortic balloon pump

f. Valvulotomy

g. Saphenous vein graft

h. Insertion of cardiac pacemaker

i. Closure of atrial septal defect

MULTIPLE CHOICE

Select the best choice to answer the question.

10. Cardiopulmonary bypass (CPB) is needed to:
    a. Oxygenate and pump the blood
    b. Wash the blood
    c. Add electrolytes to the blood
    d. All of the above

11. During cardiac surgery it is sometimes necessary to stop the heart contractions. This is done by:
    a. Infusing Lidocaine intravenously
    b. Taking the patient off the pump
    c. Providing a continuous IV drip of a neuromuscular block agent
    d. Infusing a cold cardioplegic solution into the circulatory system

12. In order to stop heart contractions, the patient must first:
    a. Be placed on CPB
    b. Have a living will in his or her chart
    c. Have the heart packed in ice
    d. Have a cardiac stabilizer put in place

13. The most common incision used for cardiac surgery is the:
    a. Anterolateral
    b. Flank
    c. Median sternotomy
    d. Subcostal

14. Coronary artery disease is associated with:
    a. Atherosclerosis
    b. Arteriosclerosis
    c. Diet and other environmental factors
    d. All of the above

15. A vacuum assisted stabilizer may be needed when:
    a. Cardioplegic solution is used
    b. The patient is placed in lateral position
    c. The heart stops during surgery
    d. The heart continues to contract during surgery

16. The purpose of a Rummel tourniquet is to:
    a. Prevent blood from flowing through an artery
    b. Retract a large nerve
    c. Retract a large artery
    d. None of the above

17. The most common site to implant a pulse battery is the:
   a. Abdomen
   b. Flank
   c. Pelvis
   d. Subclavian area

18. The function of an intra-aortic balloon catheter is to:
   a. Repair a coronary artery
   b. Repair the aortic arch
   c. Treat a problem in the conduction system
   d. Decrease the work of the heart

19. An intra-aortic balloon catheter is commonly implanted:
   a. Following a myocardial infarction
   b. Following a brain stroke
   c. In patients requiring CPB
   d. In patients awaiting a heart transplant

FILL IN THE BLANK

Fill in the blanks with the correct words.

20. The greater saphenous vein is ideal for an autograft because of these characteristics:

   a. _____

   b. _____

   c. _____

21. During closure of a median sternotomy, the surgeon may use _____ to close the sternum:

   a. _____

   b. _____

22. A fusiform aneurysm is one that _____ _____
_____.

23. A saccular aneurysm is one that _____
_____.

24. The cardiac cycle is defined as _____
_____.

25. Ventricular systole is defined as _____.

26. Diastole is defined as _____.

27. The heart is enclosed by a double layered membrane called the _____.

28. The heart muscle is called _____.

29. Valve leaflets are attached to the papillary muscle by the _____.

Label the following structures of the heart: using lines: a. R. atrium b. L. atrium c. R. ventricle d. L ventricle e. Aortic arch f. Superior vena cava g. Inferior vena cava h. Pulmonary trunk

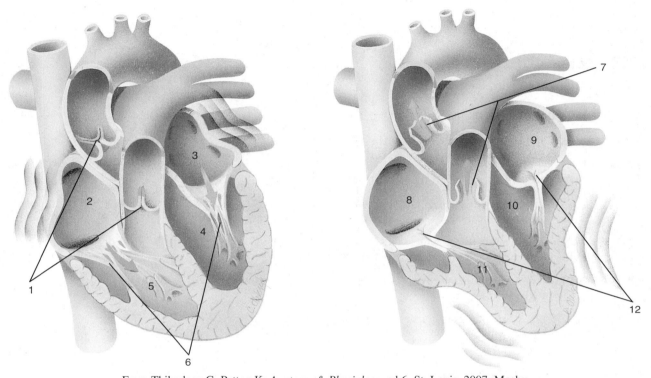

From Thibodeau G, Patton K: *Anatomy & Physiology,* ed 6, St. Louis, 2007, Mosby

34 Pediatric Surgery

MATCHING

Match the pathology with its definition.

1. _____ Malignancy of the kidney occurring in children

2. _____ Condition arising from spina bifida in which a portion of the spinal cord herniates through the skin

3. _____ A congenital separation of the hard palate

4. _____ Abdominal viscera in the fetus develops outside the body, lacking a peritoneal covering

5. _____ Congenital anomaly in which the interior surfaces of the bladder are exposed on the outer abdominal wall

6. _____ Thickening of the pyloric muscle resulting in a stricture of the proximal stomach

7. _____ A boney or membranous plate between the posterior nasal opening and the larynx

8. _____ Abdominal viscera develop in the fetus outside the body contained in a peritoneal sac

9. _____ A congenital defect in which a longitudinal groove develops in the sternum

10. _____ A congential defect that manifests as more or less than the correct number of fingers or toes

a. Gastroschisis

b. Choanal atresia

c. Omphalocele

d. Myelomeningocele

e. Cleft palate

f. Bladder exstrophy

g. Nephroblastoma

h. Pectus excavatum

i. Syndactyly

j. Pyloric stenosis

MULTIPLE CHOICE

Select one answer to complete each statement.

11. Repair of a choanal atresia may be an emergency because:
    a. The defect may bleed.
    b. The defect may cause an airway obstruction.
    c. The defect can delay development of the cranium.
    d. The defect appears at 6 months of age.

12. An infant with esophageal atresia and transesophageal atresia:
    a. Is unable to swallow nutrients
    b. May aspirate food and liquid into the lungs
    c. Often has other lethal anomalies
    d. All of the above

13. During repair of tracheoesophageal fistula:
    a. The esophagus is identified and closed with sutures.
    b. The tracheal opening is closed with sutures.
    c. The patient is placed in reverse Trendelenberg.
    d. A neck incision is used to visualize the defect.

14. In repair of omphalocele, the main objective is to:
    a. Replace all the viscera in the abdominal cavity during one procedure
    b. Suture moist towels to the skin edges
    c. Remove a portion of the intestine so the remainder can fit into the peritoneal cavity
    d. Place the viscera in a silo attached to the skin edges

15. An infant born with a gastroschisis requires emergency treatment to:
    a. Prevent the tissues from dehydration and injury
    b. Allow the infant to nurse
    c. Provide hemostasis
    d. All of the above

16. During repair of omphalocele, a _____ may be used during closure.
    a. Retention suture
    b. Autologous skin graft
    c. Mesh bridge
    d. Mesh plate

17. During orchiopexy surgery the entry incision is commonly made:
    a. Through the abdomen
    b. Through the perineum
    c. Through the base of the penis
    d. Through the external ring

18. Repair of pectus excavatum involves:
    a. Placing a bar behind the sternum
    b. Removing a portion of the midsternum
    c. Breaking the sternum
    d. Removing the entire sternum

19. During radical nephrectomy, one of the surgical goals is to:
    a. Try and salvage the diseased kidney capsule
    b. Remove the diseased kidney and its capsule
    c. Transplant the ureter of the diseased kidney to the opposite side
    d. Leave lymph nodes intact to reduce the risk of seeding

20. During surgery for syndactyly:
    a. There may be extensive bleeding
    b. Z-plasty may be necessary
    c. A rotational flap is necessary
    d. The surgeon may need to create a tunnel under the base of the thumb

FILL IN THE BLANK

Fill in the blanks with the appropriate words.

21. A parent may be allowed in the operating room during _____ to provide comfort to the child.

22. Toddlers and preschoolers believe themselves to be _____ for events in their environment.

23. Adolescent patients are very concerned about separation from their _____.

24. A _____ substance is one which causes genes to mutate, while an environmental agent or _____ causes injury to the developing fetus.

25. The word *congenital* means _____.

26. An acquired abnormality is the result of _____.

27. Lack of folic acid in the mother's diet can result in _____.

28. Herpes in the pregnant woman may result in _____ in the fetus.

29. The pediatric airway differs from the adult airway in the following ways:

    a. _____

    b. _____

    c. _____

The young pediatric patient requires specific care in the operating room during the preoperative phase. Complete the outline below to describe specific techniques required for care of the patient. Number 1 a. is given as an example.

1. Environmental factors (heat, cold, light, noise)

   a. Adjust room temperature to prevent hypothermia

   b. Prevent hyperthermia by ——

   c. Noise level —-

2. Positioning

   a.

   b.

3. Skin prep

    a.

    b.

4. Patient transport

    a.

    b.

5. Electrosurgery

    a.

    b.

6. Surgical technique

a.

b.

c.

d.

e.

35 Neurosurgery

Student's Name _____

MATCHING

Match the surgery with its objective or goal.

1. _____ Surgical entry to the cranial cavity

2. _____ Placement of a tube and reservoir to remove excess cerebrospinal fluid from the brain (hydrocephalus)

3. _____ Removal of all or part of the pituitary gland

4. _____ Removal of a cervical disk and replacement with a bone graft

5. _____ Removal of a disk and the foramen enlarged

6. _____ Mobilization of the median volar nerve from the carpel tunnel

7. _____ Creation of a section of cranium

8. _____ Use of a 3-D data map to pinpoint reference areas of the anatomy for highly accurate intervention

9. _____ Removal of a complete section of spine to include a tumor, to treat an infection, or to relieve spinal cord impingement

10. _____ Removal of prematurely fused sutures to allow expansion of the brain in the pediatric patient

a. Cervical decompression

b. Anterior cervical fusion

c. Stereotactic procedure

d. Cranioplasty

e. Ventriculoperitoneal shunt

f. Thoracic corpectomy

g. Craniotomy

h. Correction of craniosynostosis

i. Carpel tunnel release

j. Transsphenoidal hypophysectomy

MULTIPLE CHOICE

Select the best answer to complete the sentence or statement.

11. An arteriovenous fistula is:
    a. A network of arteries in the brain
    b. A network of veins in the brain
    c. Abnormal pathways between an artery and vein
    d. A feeder vessel

12. During a craniotomy the scalp is infiltrated with local anesthetic and epinephrine. This is done to:
    a. Prevent postoperative pain
    b. Expand the tissues
    c. Create tissue planes
    d. Control bleeding

13. During a craniotomy holes are drilled in the bones. This is done to:
    a. Provide a means of inserting a saw
    b. Relieve cranial pressure at the outset of the procedure
    c. Provide a means of passing instruments into the brain
    d. Control bleeding from the surface tissues

14. While the bone flap is being cut, the dura is protected from injury by the:
    a. Perforator design
    b. Raney clips
    c. Periosteal elevator
    d. Burr holes

15. Before starting the procedure for treatment of a cerebral aneurysm, the surgeon may:
    a. Test the patient's reflexes
    b. Insert a pacemaker
    c. Insert a ventricular peritoneal shunt
    d. Insert a lumbar drain

16. When positioning the patient for cerebral aneurysm surgery, the following is used:
    a. A halo vest
    b. Skin traction applied to the cervical region
    c. Cranial pin fixation
    d. An arm rest

145

17. When a cerebral aneurysm is exposed under the microscope, the scrub should have the following available:
    a. Ample bone putty to control bleeding
    b. Several suction tips
    c. Antibiotic solution
    d. An extra light source

18. Prior to surgery for arteriovenous malformation, the defect may be embolized. This is:
    a. Inserting a balloon catheter into the primary vessel
    b. Removing clots from the cerebral arteries
    c. Closing the vessels that feed the malformation
    d. Removing CSF to reduce pressure

19. In surgery to correct craniosynostosis:
    a. One or more cranial sutures are excised.
    b. A 0 degree endoscope may be needed.
    c. Bipolar ESU is used.
    d. All of the above

20. Following surgery for craniosynostosis, the child will usually be fitted for a:
    a. Mask
    b. Helmet
    c. Brace
    d. Face shield

21. A cranioplasty is performed to provide:
    a. Continuity of the cranium
    b. Protection of the brain
    c. Prevention of infection
    d. All of the above

22. In cranioplasty, the edges of the defect are trimmed in saucer shape so that:
    a. The bone cement adheres.
    b. A smooth edge is created.
    c. The scalp can be attached more easily.
    d. The prosthesis doesn't drop below the edges of the cranium.

23. When assisting in surgery for a ventriculoperitoneal shunt, the scrub must:
    a. Handle the shunt and components as little as possible
    b. Prime the assembly
    c. Have appropriate size instruments (adult or pediatric)
    d. All of the above

24. Repair of a torn nerve may be performed by joining many individual:
    a. Nerve sheaths
    b. Funiculi
    c. Neurons
    d. Axons

25. **Label as many parts as you can on this thoracic vertebra.**

_____ Vertebral foramen

_____ Epiphysis

_____ Lamina

_____ Vertebral body

_____ Costal facet

_____ Pedicle

_____ Spinous process

_____ Superior facet

_____ Transverse process

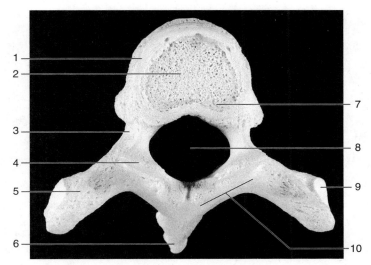

From Standring S, _Gray's Anatomy_, ed 41, Philadelphia, 2016, Elsevier

1. Ms. X is undergoing surgery for a cerebral aneurysm. The surgeon has performed a craniotomy and is ready to give you the bone flap. His request card indicates that the flap should be kept moist with saline until it is replaced at the close of the procedure. Outline the steps you will use to accept the graft, manage it, and protect it during surgery.

36 Emergency Trauma Surgery

Student's Name _____

MATCHING

Match the terms with their definition.

1. _____ Detailed assessment of the patient's injuries and physiological status

2. _____ Dysfunction of the body's clotting system

3. _____ A diagnosis confirmed by assessment or investigation

4. _____ Establishing physiologic balance in trauma

5. _____ The body's general reaction to disruption in normal homeostasis

6. _____ Exaggerated tissue swelling in a closed compartment of the body

7. _____ First rapid assessment during the prehospital phase of care

8. _____ A specific condition in which the depletion of thrombin leads to microhemorrhage and is often fatal

9. _____ Injury which is not recognized at the time of assessment

10. _____ Abnormally low blood pH and buildup of lactic acid

a. Physiological compensation

b. Secondary survey

c. Disseminated intravascular coagulation

d. Compartment syndrome

e. Occult injury

f. Definitive diagnosis

g. Metabolic acidosis

h. Coagulopathy

i. Primary survey

j. Resuscitation

MULTIPLE CHOICE

Select the best answer to the question.

11. Damage control surgery is:
    a. A procedure that protects the surgeon from lawsuit
    b. A technique in which tissues and organs are reconstructed immediately following trauma
    c. Performing surgery in the prehospital stage
    d. Life-saving surgical techniques in which reconstruction is not attempted.

12. Damage control surgery may include:
    a. Packing the wound
    b. Control of fecal spillage
    c. Reducing fractures and splinting
    d. Control of hemorrhage
    e. All of the above

13. A definitive procedure is one that is performed:
    a. During damage control surgery
    b. To secure hemostasis
    c. After the patient has been stabilized
    d. In the first 8 to 10 hours after the trauma

14. When putting together a case cart for emergency surgery, the ST should:
    a. Build upon items needed for a specific system of the body
    b. Pull instrument sets for several body systems
    c. Provide approximately 10 times the usual amount of sponges
    d. Not try to put a case cart together until he or she has spoken with the surgeon

15. Irrigation solutions used during trauma surgery should be:
    a. Cold to promote hemostasis
    b. Measured to determine blood loss
    c. Kept to a minimum to prevent DIC
    d. All of the above

16. The "lethal triangle" of physiological events includes:
    a. Hyperthermia, coagulopathy, dehydration
    b. Hematuria, coagulopathy, metabolic acidosis
    c. Coagulopathy, metabolic acidosis, hypothermia
    d. Shock, hypothermia, hemorrhage

149

17. During emergency surgery:
    a. It may not be possible to perform standard sponge counts.
    b. Sponge counts are not important.
    c. Sponge counts must be performed following standard protocol.
    d. Sponge counts are always performed at the beginning and end of the case.

18. In order to prevent bowel spillage during abdominal trauma surgery:
    a. The injured bowel will be placed in a bowel bag and repaired after 24 hours.
    b. The abdomen is thoroughly irrigated at the start of the procedure.
    c. The bowel is isolated with sponges and repaired.
    d. Isolation (bowel) technique is unnecessary because the abdomen is already contaminated.

19. A staged closure of the abdomen may require:
    a. Vacuum suction system
    b. Iodophor-impregnated drape
    c. Silastic mesh
    d. All of the above

20. Damage control orthopedic surgery often includes:
    a. Internal fixation with plates to stabilize the fracture
    b. Meticulous removal of all foreign material to prevent sepsis
    c. External fixation in the presence of extensive soft tissue damage
    d. All of the above

21. A significant priority in damage control surgery of the thorax is:
    a. Exposure to and management of hemorrhage
    b. Immediate chest wall closure and insertion of chest tubes
    c. Repair of rib fractures to prevent further injury
    d. Removal of ribs to prevent further injury

22. The most lethal complication of penetrating cardiac injury is:
    a. Cardiac tamponade
    b. Pericardial tear
    c. Flail chest
    d. Mediastinal shift

FILL IN THE BLANK

Fill in the blanks with the correct words.

23. Mechanical ventilation is necessary for a trauma patient with a(n) _____

_____ .

24. The _____ course prepares physician and non-physician treatment guidelines and protocols for trauma management.

25. Examples of blunt trauma are:

    a. _____

    b. _____

    c. _____

26. Penetrating wounds are most commonly caused by _____

_____ .

27. Thrombin-based tissue sealants are only effective when the patient has a(n) _____

_____

_____ .

SHORT ANSWER

Provide a short answer for each question or statement.

28. Explain the following: *If the problem cannot be visualized, it cannot be managed.*

_____

_____

_____

29. A *sucking* chest wound is:

_____

_____

_____

30. A *tension pneumothorax* is:

_____

_____

_____

31. Describe, in basic terms, a staged abdominal closure and the materials that might be needed.

_____

_____

_____

32. Why is external fixation using a pin and rod system often used in damage control orthopedic repair?

_____

_____

_____

33. Why is it important to avoid handling bullets and other projectiles with metal instruments?

_____

_____

_____

CASE STUDY

You are on emergency call and are directed to come to the hospital following a mass shooting. You are told on arrival that you will be scrubbing on a trauma case. The only information you have is the following:

The victim is a 32-year-old male with multiple gunshot wounds to the lower abdomen. EMTs on the scene suspected a pelvic fracture and have placed a pelvic binder on the patient. The patient's vital signs indicate hemorrhage. On arrival at the hospital, 3D CT shows a displaced fracture of the left inferior and superior rami and separation of the pubic symphysis. There also appears to be trauma at the sigmoid colon with mesenteric tearing.

1. What instruments do you need to start the case?

2. Assuming both a bowel rupture and pelvic hemorrhaging, how would you set up your instruments on the back table?

3. Do you need a clean instrument setup for bowel technique?

4. What might the priorities be for damage control surgery in this case?

Refer to the following online article from the *Journal of Orthopedic Trauma* that presents a study on gunshot wounds to the hip and pelvis:

www.ncbi.nom.nih.gov/pubmed/20871253

(Retrieved online on August 20, 2016)

Answer the questions as best you can. Remember that in a real emergency case, planning will likely be supported by experienced team members assigned to the case.

37 Disaster Preparedness

Student's Name _____

SHORT ANSWERS

Provide a short answer for each question or statement.

1. What is the difference between a disaster and an emergency?

   _____

   _____

2. List four types of weather-related disasters.

   _____

   _____

3. List four types of human-made disasters.

   _____

   _____

4. What is bioterrorism?

   _____

   _____

5. What role does the community play in disaster preparation?

   _____

   _____

6. List the primary objectives of a local disaster plan.

   _____

   _____

MATCHING

Match each term with the correct definition.

7. _____ An important activity in public health during a disaster

8. _____ Ensures that a disaster response is consistent with the doctrines and laws of the country

9. _____ A process in which people are physically moved away from the environmental dangers caused by a disaster

10. _____ A process of bringing family members in contact during and after a disaster

11. _____ Social and psychological assistance needed in every disaster

12. _____ Protects people from harsh environmental conditions

13. _____ Form the process of transport and distribution of materials, goods, food, and other necessary supplies

14. _____ A designated area for placing the dead which is removed from public areas

a. Shelter

b. Evacuation

c. Temporary morgue

d. Logistics

e. Mental health needs

f. Health messages in the community

g. Department of Homeland Security

h. Reunification

MULTIPLE CHOICE

Choose the most correct answer for each question or statement.

15. _____ is a process in which casualties are given emergency medical treatment according to the probability of their survival.
    a. Surge capacity
    b. Communication
    c. Triage
    d. Medical facility evacuation

16. A major health facility has the ability to _____ using satellite or high frequency radio.
    a. Analyze surge capacity
    b. Communicate
    c. Perform triage
    d. Evacuate injured people

17. _____ of a medical facility may sometimes be necessary because of structural hazards or immediate threat from fire, chemical, or bioterrorism.
    a. Surge capacity
    b. Communication
    c. Triage
    d. Evacuation

18. _____ is the ability of a health care facility to quickly increase its capability to receive and treat patients.
    a. Surge capacity
    b. Communication
    c. Triage
    d. Medical facility evacuation

19. Roles are assigned using a *job action sheet* (JAS). This is a tool used to define:
    a. Surge capacity
    b. Staff assignments
    c. Triage
    d. Medical facility management team

20. During a disaster, individual health care workers may be asked to:
    a. Perform tasks outside their scope of practice
    b. Perform tasks outside their usual role but within their scope of practice
    c. Perform management tasks even though they have no experience
    d. Be a spokesperson for the hospital

21. During a disaster, the press and other media require:
    a. Food and water from the health facility
    b. The ability to examine patients
    c. Lists of the dead
    d. A designated communication area for their use

CASE STUDIES

1. *Read the following scenario and answer the questions based on your knowledge of the health care disaster plan.*

   You are a CST and you are at home when a tornado hits your community.

   a. What is your first response?

   b. After you secure your family, what should you do next?

2. *Read the following scenario and answer the questions based on your knowledge of the ethical dilemmas in a disaster.*

   You are a CST working during a hurricane. You have worked over 12 hours with no breaks. Your coworkers cannot get to the hospital due to the disaster. Answer the following questions:

   a. Should you refuse to work any longer?

   b. What do you do if your husband has to have immediate surgery and there is no one there to relieve you?

   c. What are your ethical responsibilities during a disaster?

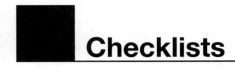

Checklists

Taking the Patient's Blood Pressure

Student's Name: _____ Date: _____

Task: Student will demonstrate the correct technique for taking a patient's blood pressure manually.

Equipment and Supplies:
- Manual blood pressure apparatus
- Stethoscope

Evaluation Directions: Place the appropriate number indicating the student's proficiency for each element using the following rating scale:

3—PROFICIENT. Can complete the task. Meets minimum entry level.

2—PARTIALLY PROFICIENT. Can complete most of the task. Needs assistance. Needs constant supervision.

1—LIMITED. Can complete a limited amount of the task. Must be told what to do. Needs extremely close supervision.

0—UNSATISFACTORY. Cannot perform the task. Lacks knowledge, skills, and critical thinking skills while performing the task.

Skills	Grade	Self-Assessment	Instructor Initial
1. Student is able to explain the purpose of taking the patient's blood pressure; knows the normal range for adults and pediatric patients.	0 1 2 3		
2. Gathers supplies, selecting the correct size blood pressure cuff.	0 1 2 3		
3. Positions patient correctly.	0 1 2 3		
4. Positions blood pressure cuff correctly on arm.	0 1 2 3		
5. Palpates the brachial artery correctly and inflates the cuff until pulse is no longer palpable. Releases cuff and waits the correct amount of time before reinflating.	0 1 2 3		
6. Places head of stethoscope over the pulse point while inflating the cuff correctly.	0 1 2 3		
7. Slowly deflates the cuff and correctly notes the levels of auscultation, including the middle level.	0 1 2 3		
8. Documents the patient's blood pressure in the patient record.	0 1 2 3		
Total			

SCORE

24	Proficient
16–23	Partially Proficient—Needs Remediation
Below 16	Unsatisfactory—Not Passing

Comments:

_____

_____

_____

_____

Student Signature: _____

Instructor Signature: _____

Measuring the Patient's Pulse

Student's Name: _____ Date: _____

Task: Student will demonstrate the correct technique for measuring and recording the patient's pulse.

Equipment and Supplies:

■ Watch or clock with second hand

Evaluation Directions: Place the appropriate number indicating the student's proficiency for each element using the following rating scale:

3—PROFICIENT. Can complete the task. Meets minimum entry level.

2—PARTIALLY PROFICIENT. Can complete most of the task. Needs assistance. Needs constant supervision.

1—LIMITED. Can complete a limited amount of the task. Must be told what to do. Needs extremely close supervision.

0—UNSATISFACTORY. Cannot perform the task. Lacks knowledge, skills, and critical thinking skills while performing the task.

Skills	Grade	Self-Assessment	Instructor Initial
1. Student is able to describe normal pulse rates for adults and children.	0 1 2 3		
2. Student can distinguish between pulse strengths and use the correct terminology in documentation.	0 1 2 3		
3. Student can explain under what circumstances the pulse is measured for 1 full minute.	0 1 2 3		
4. Student performs hand wash.	0 1 2 3		
5. Palpates the radial pulse point using correct technique.	0 1 2 3		
6. Uses watch or clock with second hand to determine the rate; measures the pulse for 1 full minute.	0 1 2 3		
7. Correctly records the pulse rate and strength in patient chart.	0 1 2 3		
Total			

SCORE

21	Proficient
13–20	Partially Proficient—Needs Remediation
Below 13	Unsatisfactory—Not Passing

Comments:

_____

_____

_____

_____

Student Signature: _____

Instructor Signature: _____

Measuring the Patient's Respiratory Rate

Student's Name: _____ Date: _____

Task: Student will demonstrate the correct technique for measuring and recording the patient's respiratory rate.

Equipment and Supplies:

■ Watch or clock with second hand.

Evaluation Directions: Place the appropriate number indicating the student's proficiency for each element using the following rating scale:

3—PROFICIENT. Can complete the task. Meets minimum entry level.

2—PARTIALLY PROFICIENT. Can complete most of the task. Needs assistance. Needs constant supervision.

1—LIMITED. Can complete a limited amount of the task. Must be told what to do. Needs extremely close supervision.

0—UNSATISFACTORY. Cannot perform the task. Lacks knowledge, skills, and critical thinking skills while performing the task.

Skills	Grade	Self-Assessment	Instructor Initial
1. Student is able to describe normal respiration rates in adults and children.	0 1 2 3		
2. Student correctly observes rise and fall of thorax and counts respirations for 1 minute.	0 1 2 3		
3. Correctly documents respiration rate in patient chart.	0 1 2 3		
Total			

SCORE

9   Proficient

6–8   Partially Proficient—Needs Remediation

Below 6   Unsatisfactory—Not Passing

Comments:

_____

_____

_____

_____

Student Signature: _____

Instructor Signature: _____

Measuring the Patient's Temperature

Student's Name: _____ Date: _____

Task: Student will demonstrate the correct technique for measuring and recording the patient's temperature.

Equipment and Supplies:
- Tympanic thermometer
- Probe covers
- Alcohol swabs

Evaluation Directions: Place the appropriate number indicating the student's proficiency for each element using the following rating scale:

3—PROFICIENT. Can complete the task. Meets minimum entry level.

2—PARTIALLY PROFICIENT. Can complete most of the task. Needs assistance. Needs constant supervision.

1—LIMITED. Can complete a limited amount of the task. Must be told what to do. Needs extremely close supervision.

0—UNSATISFACTORY. Cannot perform the task. Lacks knowledge, skills, and critical thinking skills while performing the task.

Skills	Grade	Self-Assessment	Instructor Initial
1. Student is able to describe normal temperature range and variance in temperatures among methods—oral, rectal, tympanic.	0 1 2 3		
2. Assembles supplies for taking tympanic temperature reading.	0 1 2 3		
3. Disinfects thermometer using alcohol swabs.	0 1 2 3		
4. Secures probe cover using correct technique.	0 1 2 3		
5. Uses correct technique for straightening the ear canal while inserting probe.	0 1 2 3		
6. Measures the temperature and releases probe cover into appropriate receptacle.	0 1 2 3		
7. Correctly documents temperature in patient's chart.	0 1 2 3		

SCORE

21	Proficient
14–20	Proficient—Needs Remediation
Below 14	Unsatisfactory—Not Passing

Comments:

_____

_____

_____

_____

Student Signature: _____

Instructor Signature: _____

Assessment of Technology and Equipment Skills
Compressed Gas Pneumatic Fittings and Regulator

Student's Name: _____ Date: _____

Task: Student will demonstrate the correct technique in setting up a pneumatic drill including both ends of the compressed gas (air or nitrogen) power hose including foot operated and hand operated instruments. The student must demonstrate how to use the gas regulator on a gas cylinder by pressurizing the cylinder (opening the tank) and setting the operating pressure He or she will demonstrate the instrument's safety catch. The student will demonstrate how to close the tank valve and regulator, bleed (purge) the power hose, and disconnect the hose from the compressed gas source. If a standard Schrader connector is available, this should be demonstrated.

Note: When using a compressed gas cylinder, the regulator should already be safely installed in the tank. Students should not be required to install a regulator.

Evaluation Directions: Place the appropriate number indicating the student's proficiency for each element using the following rating scale:

3—PROFICIENT. Can perform the task. Meets minimum entry level.

2—PARTIALLY PROFICIENT. Can perform most of the task. Needs assistance. Needs constant supervision.

1—LIMITED. Can do a limited amount of the task. Must be told what to do. Needs extremely close supervision.

0—UNSATISFACTORY. Cannot perform the task. Lacks knowledge, skills and critical thinking while skills performing the task.

Skills	Grade	Self-Assessment	Instructor Initial
1. Correctly and safely handles the compressed gas cylinder	0 1 2 3		
2. Correctly pressurize the cylinder regulator by opening the tank valve. Explains the minimum safe pressure in pounds per square inch (psi).	0 1 2 3		
3. Attaches the power hose to the regulator and instrument fitting. If foot controlled system is used, student should demonstrate how to connect the power hose to the foot control.	0 1 2 3		
4. Establishes the correct operating pressure for the instrument using the control knob on the regulator while instrument is running.	0 1 2 3		
5. Demonstrates the safety lock on the instrument.	0 1 2 3		
6. Demonstrates how to close the tank valve, turn the regulator pressure valve to 0 psi.	0 1 2 3		
7. Demonstrates how to purge gas from the instrument and power hose.	0 1 2 3		
8. Demonstrates how to release the power hose from the instrument and foot control, if used.			

SCORE

24	Proficient
16–23	Partially Proficient—Needs Remediation
Less than 16	Limited/Unsatisfactory—Not Passing

Comments:

_____

_____

_____

_____

Student Signature: _____

Instructor Signature: _____

Routine Hand Washing

Student's Name: _____ Date: _____

Task: Student will demonstrate the correct technique for routine hand washing.

Equipment and Supplies:

- Antiseptic soap
- Paper towels

Evaluation Directions: Place the appropriate number indicating the student's proficiency for each element using the following rating scale:

3—PROFICIENT. Can complete the task. Meets minimum entry level.

2—PARTIALLY PROFICIENT. Can complete most of the task. Needs assistance. Needs constant supervision.

1—LIMITED. Can complete a limited amount of the task. Must be told what to do. Needs extremely close supervision.

0—UNSATISFACTORY. Cannot perform the task. Lacks knowledge, skills, and critical thinking skills while performing the task.

Skills	Grade	Self-Assessment	Instructor Initial
1. Correctly describes the purpose and importance of frequent hand washing.	0 1 2 3		
2. Prepares for task: jewelry removed and scrub top tucked in.	0 1 2 3		
3. Washes all areas of both hands and wrists correctly.	0 1 2 3		
4. Rinses hands and wrists thoroughly, holding fingertips down.	0 1 2 3		
5. Prevents scrub clothes from touching sink or being splashed with water during procedure.	0 1 2 3		
6. Dries hands thoroughly with paper towel and disposes of towel.	0 1 2 3		
7. Uses a clean, dry towel to turn water off.	0 1 2 3		
Total			

SCORE

21	Proficient
14–20	Partially Proficient—Needs Remediation
Below 14	Unsatisfactory—Not Passing

Comments:

_____

_____

_____

_____

Student Signature: _____

Instructor Signature: _____

Surgical Scrub

Student's Name: _____ Date: _____

Task: Student will demonstrate the correct technique for the traditional surgical scrub.

Equipment and Supplies:

- Antiseptic soap
- Sterile scrub sponges
- Nail cleaners
- Surgical mask
- Protective eyewear or face shield

Evaluation Directions: Place the appropriate number indicating the student's proficiency for each element using the following rating scale:

3—PROFICIENT. Can complete the task. Meets minimum entry level.

2—PARTIALLY PROFICIENT. Can complete most of the task. Needs assistance. Needs constant supervision.

1—LIMITED. Can complete a limited amount of the task. Must be told what to do. Needs extremely close supervision.

0—UNSATISFACTORY. Cannot perform the task. Lacks knowledge, skills, and critical thinking skills while performing the task.

Skills	Grade	Self-Assessment	Instructor Initial
1. Is able to explain the purpose of the task and principles of aseptic technique involved.	0 1 2 3		
2. Prepares for task: dons face mask and protective eyewear or face shield.	0 1 2 3		
3. Prepares for task: tucks in scrub top and scrub pants ties.	0 1 2 3		
4. Prepares for task: removes all jewelry.	0 1 2 3		
5. Sweeps all subungual areas with plastic nail cleaner under running water. Discards nail cleaner appropriately.	0 1 2 3		
6. Using sterile presoaped scrub sponge, washes fingertips and nails by passing them back and forth across the sponge. *Timed method:* 2 minutes per hand. *Stroke method:* 30 strokes per hand.	0 1 2 3		
7. Washes 4 sides of each finger and between the finger webs. *Timed method:* 2 minutes per hand. *Stroke method:* 10 strokes for each side of each finger and thumb.	0 1 2 3		
8. Washes the dorsal and palm sides of each hand. *Timed method:* 1 minute per hand. *Stroke method:* 30 strokes for each side of the hand.	0 1 2 3		

Continued

Skills	Grade	Self-Assessment	Instructor Initial
9. Washes the four sides of wrists and forearms in circular pattern to 2" above the elbows. *Timed method:* 1 minute for each arm. *Stroke method:* 10 strokes for each of four planes.	0 1 2 3		
10. Discards sponge in appropriate receptacle.	0 1 2 3		
11. Rinses hands and arms with hands and arms held higher than elbows; allows running water to flow from hands to arms only.	0 1 2 3		
12. In the event any part of the hand or arm touches the faucet or sink, student knows to repeat the scrub process on that area.	0 1 2 3		
13. Proceeds to the operating room with elbows flexed; backs through the OR door.	0 1 2 3		
Total			

SCORE

39	Proficient
26–39	Partially Proficient—Needs Remediation
Below 26	Unsatisfactory—Not Passing

Comments:

_____

_____

_____

_____

Student Signature: _____

Instructor Signature: _____

Surgical Hand and Arm Antisepsis

Student's Name: _____ Date: _____

Task: Student will demonstrate the correct technique for performing a hand and arm rub.

Equipment and Supplies:

- Surgical grade antiseptic
- Face mask
- Protective eyewear

Evaluation Directions: Place the appropriate number indicating the student's proficiency for each element using the following rating scale:

3—PROFICIENT. Can complete the task. Meets minimum entry level.

2—PARTIALLY PROFICIENT. Can complete most of the task. Needs assistance. Needs constant supervision.

1—LIMITED. Can complete a limited amount of the task. Must be told what to do. Needs extremely close supervision.

0—UNSATISFACTORY. Cannot perform the task. Lacks knowledge, skills, and critical thinking skills while performing the task.

Skills	Grade	Self-Assessment	Instructor Initial
1. Is able to explain the purpose of the skill, including under what circumstances a hand and arm rub should be used.	0 1 2 3		
2. Prepares for task: dons face mask and protective eyewear.	0 1 2 3		
3. Prepares for task: tucks in scrub top and scrub pants ties.	0 1 2 3		
4. Prepares for task: removes all jewelry.	0 1 2 3		
5. Follows manufacturer's recommendations for amount of antiseptic to use and dispenses only this amount into one hand.	0 1 2 3		
6. Sweeps fingertips of opposite hand in a circular motion through the antiseptic.	0 1 2 3		
7. Spreads antiseptic to entire hand, including finger webs.	0 1 2 3		
8. Spreads antiseptic to forearm and elbow, covering all surfaces in a circular motion.	0 1 2 3		
9. Repeats the process on the opposite hand and arm.	0 1 2 3		
10. Dispenses 2 to 5 mL of antiseptic into one hand.	0 1 2 3		
11. Rubs palms together to distribute antiseptic to both hands.	0 1 2 3		

Continued

Skills	Grade	Self-Assessment	Instructor Initial
12. Places the palm of one hand over the back of the other and interlaces the fingers. Passes the top hand back and forth over the bottom hand to cleanse the webs. Reverses the position of the hands and repeats the process.	0 1 2 3		
13. Holds the fingertips of each hand in the palm of the other hand and moves the fingertips back and forth.	0 1 2 3		
14. Cleanses the webs of each thumb by clasping it in the opposite hand and rubbing.	0 1 2 3		
15. Completes the procedure in the time recommended by the manufacturer of the antiseptic.	0 1 2 3		
Total			

SCORE

45	Proficient
30–44	Partially Proficient—Needs Remediation
Below 30	Unsatisfactory—Not Passing

Comments:

_____

_____

_____

_____

Student Signature: _____

Instructor Signature: _____

Drying the Hands and Arms Aseptically

Student's Name: _____ Date: _____

Task: Student will demonstrate the correct technique for drying the hands and arms following the surgical scrub (scrub role).

Equipment and Supplies:

■ Gown pack with sterile towel

Evaluation Directions: Place the appropriate number indicating the student's proficiency for each element using the following rating scale:

3—PROFICIENT. Can complete the task. Meets minimum entry level.

2—PARTIALLY PROFICIENT. Can complete most of the task. Needs assistance. Needs constant supervision.

1—LIMITED. Can complete a limited amount of the task. Must be told what to do. Needs extremely close supervision.

0—UNSATISFACTORY. Cannot perform the task. Lacks knowledge, skills, and critical thinking skills while performing the task.

Skills	Grade	Self-Assessment	Instructor Initial
1. Able to explain the purpose of the skill.	0 1 2 3		
2. Maintains hands above elbows while approaching the gown and towel pack.	0 1 2 3		
3. Grasps the towel and moves it cleanly up and away from the gown.	0 1 2 3		
4. Prevents water from dripping onto the sterile gown.	0 1 2 3		
5. While bending at the waist suspends one end of the towel, allowing it to unfold lengthwise between his or her two hands.	0 1 2 3		
6. Confines one hand on one towel surface and the other hand on the other towel surface. Blots the skin, moving from hand to wrist to arm.	0 1 2 3		
7. Prevents contamination of the towel by the scrub suit.	0 1 2 3		
8. Places the other hand at the opposite end of the towel and repeats the blotting process on that hand and arm.	0 1 2 3		
9. Drops the towel in an appropriate receptacle when finished.	0 1 2 3		
Total			

SCORE

27	Proficient
18–26	Partially Proficient—Needs Remediation
Below 18	Unsatisfactory—Not Passing

Comments:

_____

_____

_____

_____

Student Signature: _____

Instructor Signature: _____

Unassisted Gowning and Gloving

Student's Name: _____ Date: _____

Task: Student will demonstrate the correct technique for self-gowning and gloving in the scrub role.

Equipment and Supplies:
- Sterile gown
- Sterile gloves

Evaluation Directions: Place the appropriate number indicating the student's proficiency for each element using the following rating scale:

3—PROFICIENT. Can complete the task. Meets minimum entry level.

2—PARTIALLY PROFICIENT. Can complete most of the task. Needs assistance. Needs constant supervision.

1—LIMITED. Can complete a limited amount of the task. Must be told what to do. Needs extremely close supervision.

0—UNSATISFACTORY. Cannot perform the task. Lacks knowledge, skills, and critical thinking skills while performing the task.

Skills	Grade	Self-Assessment	Instructor Initial
1. Able to explain the principles and purpose of self-gowning and gloving.	0 1 2 3		
2. Grasps the folded gown below the neckline without touching the front of the gown.	0 1 2 3		
3. Lifts the entire folded gown up and away from the table cleanly.	0 1 2 3		
4. Allows the gown to unfold with the outside surface facing away. Maintains grasp at the neckline.	0 1 2 3		
5. Identifies the armholes and advances the hands and arms through the sleeves, stopping at the point where the cuffs attach to the sleeve (cuff seam).	0 1 2 3		
6. Enables nonsterile person to secure neck and back ties.	0 1 2 3		
7. Keeping the hands well inside the gown sleeve, correctly positions the glove palm to palm and glove cuff to sleeve cuff.	0 1 2 3		
8. Demonstrates proficiency in keeping the fingertips back and away from the cuff edges while flipping and pulling the glove over the cuff and sleeve.	0 1 2 3		
9. Gently advances the fingers and hand into the glove while keeping the gown cuff completely covered by the glove.	0 1 2 3		
10. Repeats the process to glove the other hand.	0 1 2 3		
11. Demonstrates proficiency in turning the gown with nonsterile person.	0 1 2 3		
Total			

SCORE

33	Proficient
22–32	Partially Proficient—Needs Remediation
Below 22	Unsatisfactory—Not Passing

Comments:

_____

_____

_____

_____

Student Signature: _____

Instructor Signature: _____

Opening Sterile Instrument Tray

Student's Name: _____ Date: _____

Task: Student will demonstrate the correct technique for opening a wrapped instrument tray on a small table in the circulator role.

Equipment and Supplies:

- Large instrument tray wrapped envelope style
- Small table

Evaluation Directions: Place the appropriate number indicating the student's proficiency for each element using the following rating scale:

3—PROFICIENT. Can complete the task. Meets minimum entry level.

2—PARTIALLY PROFICIENT. Can complete most of the task. Needs assistance. Needs constant supervision.

1—LIMITED. Can complete a limited amount of the task. Must be told what to do. Needs extremely close supervision.

0—UNSATISFACTORY. Cannot perform the task. Lacks knowledge, skills, and critical thinking skills while performing the task.

Skills	Grade	Self-Assessment	Instructor Initial
1. Is able to explain the rationale for the technique used in this skill.	0 1 2 3		
2. Places wrapped instrument tray in the correct orientation on the table.	0 1 2 3		
3. Checks indicator tape for color change and inspects the outside for watermarks or holes.	0 1 2 3		
4. Breaks the tape to release the first flap of the cover.	0 1 2 3		
5. Grasps the edge of the first flap on the far side of the tray and pulls it back and away.	0 1 2 3		
6. Grasps one of the side flaps by the edge and pulls it away and down. Repeats process on second side flap.	0 1 2 3		
7. Grasps the nearest flap by the edge and pulls it away while stepping back away from the table.	0 1 2 3		
8. Avoids leaning into the tray or reaching over the exposed sterile surface at any time during opening.	0 1 2 3		
9. Maintains safe distance of 12 inches from the sterile tray during opening.	0 1 2 3		
Total			

SCORE

27	Proficient
18–26	Partially Proficient—Needs Remediation
Below 18	Unsatisfactory—Not Passing

Comments:

_____

_____

_____

_____

Student Signature: _____

Instructor Signature: _____

Opening Sterile Basins

Student's Name: _____ Date: _____

Task: Student will demonstrate the correct technique for opening a sterile basin positioned in a ring stand. The nonsterile role is to be demonstrated.

Equipment and Supplies:

- Ring stand
- Wrapped sterile basin

Evaluation Directions: Place the appropriate number indicating the student's proficiency for each element using the following rating scale:

3—PROFICIENT. Can complete the task. Meets minimum entry level.

2—PARTIALLY PROFICIENT. Can complete most of the task. Needs assistance. Needs constant supervision.

1—LIMITED. Can complete a limited amount of the task. Must be told what to do. Needs extremely close supervision.

0—UNSATISFACTORY. Cannot perform the task. Lacks knowledge, skills, and critical thinking skills while performing the task.

Skills	Grade	Self-Assessment	Instructor Initial
1. Student is able to explain the rationale for the sterile technique used in this skill.	0 1 2 3		
2. Student positions the wrapped basin in the ring stand so that the first flap of the wrapper to be opened is on the far side.	0 1 2 3		
3. Checks the external process monitor on the basin wrapper.	0 1 2 3		
4. Checks the wrapper for watermarks, holes, or tears.	0 1 2 3		
5. Grasps the corner of the flap on the far side of the basin and pulls it away from the basin and down.	0 1 2 3		
6. Pulls the side flaps back and down.	0 1 2 3		
7. Pulls the near (last) flap away from the basin and down.	0 1 2 3		
8. Maintains a safe distance from the wrapped basin throughout the procedure.	0 1 2 3		
Total			

SCORE

24	Proficient
16–23	Partially Proficient—Needs Remediation
Below 16	Unsatisfactory—Not Passing

Comments:

_____

_____

_____

_____

Student Signature: _____

Instructor Signature: _____

Removing Contaminated Glove

Student's Name: _____ Date: _____

Task: Student will demonstrate the correct technique used by a nonsterile team member to remove the contaminated glove of a sterile team member.

Equipment and Supplies:

■ Gowned and gloved sterile team member

Evaluation Directions: Place the appropriate number indicating the student's proficiency for each element using the following rating scale:

3—PROFICIENT. Can complete the task. Meets minimum entry level.

2—PARTIALLY PROFICIENT. Can complete most of the task. Needs assistance. Needs constant supervision.

1—LIMITED. Can complete a limited amount of the task. Must be told what to do. Needs extremely close supervision.

0—UNSATISFACTORY. Cannot perform the task. Lacks knowledge, skills, and critical thinking skills while performing the task.

Skills	Grade	Self-Assessment	Instructor Initial
1. The student can explain the rationale for techniques used in this skill.	0 1 2 3		
2. The student dons nonsterile gloves.	0 1 2 3		
3. A sterile team member presents the contaminated hand to the student.	0 1 2 3		
4. The student grasps *only* the glove palm and back, not the gown cuff.	0 1 2 3		
5. The student pulls the glove off the hand of the sterile team member cleanly, without allowing it to snap back.	0 1 2 3		
6. The student discards glove in the correct receptacle.	0 1 2 3		
Total			

SCORE

18	Proficient
12–17	Partially Proficient—Needs Remediation
Below 12	Unsatisfactory—Not Passing

Comments:

_____

_____

_____

_____

Student Signature: _____

Instructor Signature: _____

Removing Gown and Gloves from Another

Student's Name: _____ Date: _____

Task: Student will demonstrate the correct technique required for a nonsterile team member to remove the gown and gloves of a sterile team member. Under normal circumstances, the surgical technologist performs self-gowning and gloving but gowns and gloves the surgeons as needed.

Equipment and Supplies:

■ Gown and gloves

Evaluation Directions: Place the appropriate number indicating the student's proficiency for each element using the following rating scale:

3—PROFICIENT. Can complete the task. Meets minimum entry level.

2—PARTIALLY PROFICIENT. Can complete most of the task. Needs assistance. Needs constant supervision.

1—LIMITED. Can complete a limited amount of the task. Must be told what to do. Needs extremely close supervision.

0—UNSATISFACTORY. Cannot perform the task. Lacks knowledge, skills, and critical thinking skills while performing the task.

Skills	Grade	Self-Assessment	Instructor Initial
1. Student understands the rationale for the techniques used in the skill and can explain under what circumstances the skill is required.	0 1 2 3		
2. Student opens a sterile gown and gloves on a small table near the sterile field.	0 1 2 3		
3. Student dons nonsterile gloves and releases the back ties of the sterile team member's gown. The sterile team member releases the side tie of the gown.	0 1 2 3		
4. Grasping the gown below the shoulders, the student pulls it away from the sterile team member's body and hands. He or she gathers the gown inward to avoid touching the contaminated side and discards the gown in the appropriate receptacle.	0 1 2 3		
5. The nonsterile team member removes the sterile team member's gloves using the technique described in *Removing a Contaminated Glove*. He or she discards the gloves in the appropriate receptacle.	0 1 2 3		
6. The sterile team member proceeds with self-gowning and gloving using closed technique or is gowned and gloved by another sterile team member.	0 1 2 3		
7. The nonsterile student secures the back ties of the sterile gown and assists in turning the flap.	0 1 2 3		
Total			

SCORE

21	Proficient
14–20	Partially Proficient—Needs Remediation
Below 14	Unsatisfactory—Not Passing

Comments:

_____

_____

_____

_____

Student Signature: _____

Instructor Signature: _____

Assisted Gowning and Gloving

Student's Name: _____ Date: _____

Task: Student will demonstrate the correct technique for gowning and gloving the surgeon.

Equipment and Supplies:
- Gowns and gloves for two people
- Table with sterile cover

Evaluation Directions: Place the appropriate number indicating the student's proficiency for each element using the following rating scale:

3—PROFICIENT. Can complete the task. Meets minimum entry level.

2—PARTIALLY PROFICIENT. Can complete most of the task. Needs assistance. Needs constant supervision.

1—LIMITED. Can complete a limited amount of the task. Must be told what to do. Needs extremely close supervision.

0—UNSATISFACTORY. Cannot perform the task. Lacks knowledge, skills, and critical thinking skills while performing the task.

Skills	Grade	Self-Assessment	Instructor Initial
1. The student is able to explain the rationale for techniques required in the skill.	0 1 2 3		
2. After gowning and gloving self, the student scrub removes a sterile gown from the table.	0 1 2 3		
3. Facing the other sterile team member (surgeon), he or she orients the folded gown so that the inside face is closest to the surgeon.	0 1 2 3		
4. The student grasps the gown below the shoulder and neck line, forming a cuff over his or her gloved hands, and allows the gown to unfold naturally.	0 1 2 3		
5. As the surgeon steps forward, placing the arms into the sleeves, the student must continue to hold the gown steady.	0 1 2 3		
6. The student must avoid raising his or her arms to drape the gown over the surgeon's shoulders.	0 1 2 3		
7. A nonsterile team member (circulator) pulls the gown up and over the shoulders of the surgeon and secures the neck and back ties.	0 1 2 3		
8. The student retracts the sleeves to expose the surgeon's hands.	0 1 2 3		
9. The student takes the right hand glove from its wrapper and orients it so that the palm of the glove faces the surgeon.	0 1 2 3		

Continued

Skills	Grade	Self-Assessment	Instructor Initial
10. The student places both hands under the glove cuff and stretches it open. The surgeon places his or her hand inside the glove. At the same time, the student pulls the glove over the surgeon's hand and wrist to completely cover the gown cuff.	0 1 2 3		
11. The student gloves the surgeon's other hand using the same technique.	0 1 2 3		
12. The student gloves the surgeon with the second pair of gloves using the same technique.	0 1 2 3		
Total			

SCORE

36	Proficient
24–35	Partially Proficient—Needs Remediation
Below 24	Unsatisfactory—Not Passing

Comments:

_____

_____

_____

_____

Student Signature: _____

Instructor Signature: _____

Scrub Attire

Student's Name: _____ Date: _____

Task: Student will demonstrate the correct technique for donning scrub attire, including cap and mask. Student may don a scrub suit, cap, and mask, and report to the instructor for assessment and discussion.

Equipment and Supplies:

- Scrub suit or dress
- Cap
- Mask

Evaluation Directions: Place the appropriate number indicating the student's proficiency for each element using the following rating scale:

3—PROFICIENT. Can complete the task. Meets minimum entry level.

2—PARTIALLY PROFICIENT. Can complete most of the task. Needs assistance. Needs constant supervision.

1—LIMITED. Can complete a limited amount of the task. Must be told what to do. Needs extremely close supervision.

0—UNSATISFACTORY. Cannot perform the task. Lacks knowledge, skills, and critical thinking skills while performing the task.

Skills	Grade	Self-Assessment	Instructor Initial
1. The student is able to explain the rationale for donning a freshly laundered scrub suit each day, and the reason why the surgical cap is donned before all other pieces of the scrub attire.	0 1 2 3		
2. The student's fingernails are without paint or extensions. Their length is ¼" or less.	0 1 2 3		
3. The student has selected an appropriate size scrub suit.	0 1 2 3		
4. The student has ensured that the entire hairline (men and women) is concealed behind the cap.	0 1 2 3		
5. The male student has donned a beard cover as necessary to cover all facial hair.	0 1 2 3		
6. The student has removed any jewelry that is not concealed by scrub attire, including body piercing jewelry.	0 1 2 3		
7. If the student is wearing an undershirt under the scrub top, it is completely concealed under the scrub attire.	0 1 2 3		
8. The scrub top is tucked into the scrub pants, and the pant ties are tucked into the pants	0 1 2 3		
9. The student's ID badge is pinned to the scrub top.	0 1 2 3		
10. The student has donned a freshly laundered cover jacket supplied by the facility.	0 1 2 3		

Continued

Skills	Grade	Self-Assessment	Instructor Initial
11. The student has donned shoes appropriate to the surgical environment and dedicated for that use only, or concealed by shoe covers.	0 1 2 3		
12. The student has secured the surgical cap with one tie near the crown of the head and the other at the neck. The nasal piece has been flexed over the bridge of the nose.	0 1 2 3		
Total			

SCORE

36   Proficient

24–35   Partially Proficient—Needs Remediation

Below 24   Unsatisfactory—Not Passing

Comments:

_____

_____

_____

_____

Student Signature: _____

Instructor Signature: _____

Managing Irrigation Solutions

Student's Name: _____ Date: _____

Task: Student will demonstrate the correct technique for receiving irrigation solutions and filling irrigation devices.

Equipment and Supplies:

- Gown and gloves
- Ring stand
- Basin pack
- Asepto syringe
- Bulb syringe
- Medication labels and fine tip marker

Evaluation Directions: Place the appropriate number indicating the student's proficiency for each element using the following rating scale:

3—PROFICIENT. Can perform the task. Meets minimum entry level.

2—PARTIALLY PROFICIENT. Can perform most of the task. Needs assistance. Needs constant supervision.

1—LIMITED. Can do a limited amount of the task. Must be told what to do. Needs extremely close supervision.

0—UNSATISFACTORY. Cannot perform the task. Lacks knowledge, skills, and critical thinking skills while performing the task.

Skills	Grade	Self-Assessment	Instructor Initial
1. Student correctly receives irrigation solution from circulator using protocol for visual and verbal assessment of the solution, identification, and strength.	0 1 2 3		
2. Circulator pours solution into basin using aseptic technique; student and circulator again identify the name of the solution and its strength.	0 1 2 3		
3. Student correctly labels the solution.	0 1 2 3		
4. Student fills asepto syringe correctly.	0 1 2 3		
5. Fills bulb syringe correctly.	0 1 2 3		
6. Circulator maintains solution container in the room during the surgery.	0 1 2 3		
Total			

SCORE

18	Proficient
12–17	Partially Proficient—Needs Remediation
Below 12	Unsatisfactory—Not Passing

Comments:

_____

_____

_____

_____

Student Signature: _____

Instructor Signature: _____

Room Turnover

Student's Name: _____ Date: _____

Task: Student will demonstrate the correct technique for room turnover after surgery.

Equipment and Supplies:

- Disinfectants
- Clean mop
- Wet vacuum
- Cleaning supplies

Evaluation Directions: Place the appropriate number indicating the student's proficiency for each element using the following rating scale:

3—PROFICIENT. Can perform the task. Meets minimum entry level.

2—PARTIALLY PROFICIENT. Can perform most of the task. Needs assistance. Needs constant supervision.

1—LIMITED. Can do a limited amount of the task. Must be told what to do. Needs extremely close supervision.

0—UNSATISFACTORY. Cannot perform the task. Lacks knowledge, skills, and critical thinking skills while performing the task.

Skill	Grade	Self-Assessment	Instructor Initial
1. Student removes pads from the OR table, exposing the hard surface of the table.	0 1 2 3		
2. Cleans all surfaces of table, including hinges, pivotal points, and castors	0 1 2 3		
3. Moves OR table aside; checks for any items dropped during surgery.	0 1 2 3		
4. Mops or wet vacuums underneath table, including a 3 to 4 ft. area around the table.	0 1 2 3		
5. Cleans all soiled OR equipment with disinfectant.	0 1 2 3		
6. Spot cleans walls, doors, surgical lights, ceiling supply cabinet doors, latches, and handles.	0 1 2 3		
7. Removes all contaminated items used during cleaning process from room.	0 1 2 3		
8. Repositions furniture.	0 1 2 3		
9. Places clean linen on OR table.	0 1 2 3		
10. Places liner bags in kick buckets and other receptacles.	0 1 2 3		
Total			

SCORE

30	Proficient
20–29	Partially Proficient—Needs Remediation
Below 20	Unsatisfactory—Not Passing

Comments:

_____

_____

_____

_____

Student Signature: _____

Instructor Signature: _____

SKILLS PERFORMANCE CHECKLIST—CHAPTER 10

Hand Cleaning Instruments

Student's Name: _____ Date: _____

Task: Student will demonstrate the correct technique for cleaning instruments by hand.

Equipment and Supplies:

- PPE
- Instrument set
- Enzymatic cleaner
- Detergent
- Instrument brushes and stylets
- Basins
- Syringes, size 30
- Distilled water

Evaluation Directions: Place the appropriate number indicating the student's proficiency for each element using the following rating scale:

3—PROFICIENT. Can perform the task. Meets minimum entry level.

2—PARTIALLY PROFICIENT. Can perform most of the task. Needs assistance. Needs constant supervision.

1—LIMITED. Can do a limited amount of the task. Must be told what to do. Needs extremely close supervision.

0—UNSATISFACTORY. Cannot perform the task. Lacks knowledge, skills, and critical thinking skills while performing the task.

Skills	Grade	Self-Assessment	Instructor Initial
1. Student dons correct PPE attire.	0 1 2 3		
2. Prepares enzymatic solution, detergent, brushes, stylets, and other cleaning supplies.	0 1 2 3		
3. Sorts instruments correctly, disassembling those with parts; opens all instruments.	0 1 2 3		
4. Rinses instruments with cool water.	0 1 2 3		
5. Prepares enzymatic soaking solutions for each group of instruments according to the manufacturer's recommendations. Soaks instruments for 10 minutes.	0 1 2 3		
6. Using brushes and stylets, cleans instruments under water line.	0 1 2 3		
7. Shows attention to hard to reach areas including box locks, ridges, rasp teeth, and tips.	0 1 2 3		
8. Rinses instruments, instrument channels, and hollow tubes thoroughly with distilled water.	0 1 2 3		
9. Cleans nonimmersible instruments according to manufacturer's recommendations.	0 1 2 3		
Total			

SCORE

27	Proficient
18–26	Partially Proficient—Needs Remediation
Below 18	Unsatisfactory—Not Passing

Comments:

_____

_____

_____

_____

Student Signature: _____

Instructor Signature: _____

Assemble Instrument Set

Student's Name: _____ Date: _____

Task: Student will demonstrate the correct technique for assembling an instrument set.

Equipment and Supplies:
- Clean instrument set
- Instrument sterilization tray
- Towels
- Count sheet
- Instrument stringer
- Instrument tip protectors
- Process indicators

Evaluation Directions: Place the appropriate number indicating the student's proficiency for each element using the following rating scale:

3—PROFICIENT. Can perform the task. Meets minimum entry level.

2—PARTIALLY PROFICIENT. Can perform most of the task. Needs assistance. Needs constant supervision.

1—LIMITED. Can do a limited amount of the task. Must be told what to do. Needs extremely close supervision.

0—UNSATISFACTORY. Cannot perform the task. Lacks knowledge, skills, and critical thinking skills while performing the task.

Skills	Grade	Self-Assessment	Instructor Initial
1. Student dons correct attire including long-sleeved cover jacket.	0 1 2 3		
2. Student obtains count sheet from workroom files.	0 1 2 3		
3. Organizes instruments into categories on clean work table.	0 1 2 3		
4. Prepares sterilization tray, towel liner, and stringer correctly.	0 1 2 3		
5. Inspects all instruments to ensure they are free of any debris; inspects all instruments for damage.	0 1 2 3		
6. Using a count sheet, selects the correct instruments and places them correctly in order on the stringer.	0 1 2 3		
7. Places instruments on stringer in tray, ensuring that tips are not caught in tray perforations; places tip protectors on pointed clamps and sharps.	0 1 2 3		
8. Flushes a small amount of distilled water through each suction tip.	0 1 2 3		
9. According to facility policy, places all remaining instruments in tray.	0 1 2 3		
10. Places process indicator in tray.	0 1 2 3		
Total			

SCORE

30	Proficient
20–29	Partially Proficient—Needs Remediation
Below 20	Unsatisfactory—Not Passing

Comments:

_____

_____

_____

_____

Student Signature: _____

Instructor Signature: _____

Wrapping Instruments in Peel Pouches

Student's Name: _____ Date: _____

Task: Student will demonstrate the correct technique for wrapping instruments in a peel pouch.

Equipment and Supplies:

- Peel pouch system
- Instruments for wrapping
- Process indicators
- Run stickers
- Marker

Evaluation Directions: Place the appropriate number indicating the student's proficiency for each element using the following rating scale:

3—PROFICIENT. Can perform the task. Meets minimum entry level.

2—PARTIALLY PROFICIENT. Can perform most of the task. Needs assistance. Needs constant supervision.

1—LIMITED. Can do a limited amount of the task. Must be told what to do. Needs extremely close supervision.

0—UNSATISFACTORY. Cannot perform the task. Lacks knowledge, skills, and critical thinking skills while performing the task.

Skills	Grade	Self-Assessment	Instructor Initial
1. Student dons correct attire, including long-sleeved cover jacket.	0 1 2 3		
2. Student correctly prepares instrument(s) for wrapping, including tip protectors as needed; opens instrument(s).	0 1 2 3		
3. Selects the correct size pouch for instrument(s).	0 1 2 3		
4. If using continuous roll, cuts the correct size section and seals one end correctly.	0 1 2 3		
5. Places instrument inside pouch with process indicator.	0 1 2 3		
6. Removes excess air from pouch and seals it correctly	0 1 2 3		
7. Places outside process indicator and run sticker; labels the pouch with marker.	0 1 2 3		
Total			

SCORE

21   Proficient

14–20   Partially Proficient—Needs Remediation

Below 14   Unsatisfactory—Not Passing

Comments:

_____

_____

_____

_____

Student Signature: _____

Instructor Signature: _____

Wrapping Items Envelope Style

Student's Name: _____ Date: _____

Task: Student will demonstrate the correct technique for wrapping items for sterilization using envelope style.

Equipment and Supplies:

- Instrument tray
- Wrapping material—bonded synthetic or linen
- Process indicators internal and external
- Run labels

Evaluation Directions: Place the appropriate number indicating the student's proficiency for each element using the following rating scale:

3—PROFICIENT. Can perform the task. Meets minimum entry level.

2—PARTIALLY PROFICIENT. Can perform most of the task. Needs assistance. Needs constant supervision.

1—LIMITED. Can do a limited amount of the task. Must be told what to do. Needs extremely close supervision.

0—UNSATISFACTORY. Cannot perform the task. Lacks knowledge, skills, and critical thinking skills while performing the task.

Skills	Grade	Self-Assessment	Instructor Initial
1. Student dons correct attire, including long-sleeved cover jacket.	0 1 2 3		
2. Selects the correct size wrapping material.	0 1 2 3		
3. Ensures that process indicator is included in tray.	0 1 2 3		
4. Correctly wraps the item, ensuring there are no gaps.	0 1 2 3		
5. Places external process indicator tape securely and labels the item correctly.	0 1 2 3		
6. Places run sticker on item.	0 1 2 3		
Total			

SCORE

18	Proficient
12–17	Partially Proficient—Needs Remediation
Below 12	Unsatisfactory—Not Passing

Comments:

_____

_____

_____

_____

Student Signature: _____

Instructor Signature: _____

Rigid Sterilization Container

Student's Name: _____ Date: _____

Task: Student will demonstrate the correct technique when preparing instruments for sterilization using a rigid sterilization container.

Equipment and Supplies:

- Assembled instrument tray
- Rigid sterilization system
- Filters
- Process indicators
- Tamper-proof locks

Evaluation Directions: Place the appropriate number indicating the student's proficiency for each element using the following rating scale:

3—PROFICIENT. Can perform the task. Meets minimum entry level.

2—PARTIALLY PROFICIENT. Can perform most of the task. Needs assistance. Needs constant supervision.

1—LIMITED. Can do a limited amount of the task. Must be told what to do. Needs extremely close supervision.

0—UNSATISFACTORY. Cannot perform the task. Lacks knowledge, skills, and critical thinking skills while performing the task.

Skills	Grade	Self-Assessment	Instructor Initial
1. Student dons correct attire, including long-sleeved cover jacket.	0 1 2 3		
2. Student selects the correct size container for instrument tray.	0 1 2 3		
3. Correctly inserts container filters and plates.	0 1 2 3		
4. Places internal process monitor in instrument tray.	0 1 2 3		
5. Places instrument tray inside sterilization container	0 1 2 3		
6. Correctly fits container lid and closes latches; correctly places one tamper-proof lock on each latch.	0 1 2 3		
7. Places process indicator tape and run sticker on container lid; labels the container correctly.	0 1 2 3		
Total			

SCORE

21	Proficient
14–20	Partially Proficient—Needs Remediation
Below 14	Unsatisfactory—Not Passing

Comments:

_____

_____

_____

_____

Student Signature: _____

Instructor Signature: _____

Wrapping Items Using Square Wrap

Student's Name: _____ Date: _____

Task: Student will demonstrate the correct technique for wrapping items using square wrap technique.

Equipment and Supplies:

- Prepared item to be wrapped
- Wrapping material—bonded synthetic or woven wraps
- Process indicators
- Run stickers
- Marker

Evaluation Directions: Place the appropriate number indicating the student's proficiency for each element using the following rating scale:

3—PROFICIENT. Can perform the task. Meets minimum entry level.

2—PARTIALLY PROFICIENT. Can perform most of the task. Needs assistance. Needs constant supervision.

1—LIMITED. Can do a limited amount of the task. Must be told what to do. Needs extremely close supervision.

0—UNSATISFACTORY. Cannot perform the task. Lacks knowledge, skills, and critical thinking skills while performing the task.

Skills	Grade	Self-Assessment	Instructor Initial
1. Student dons correct attire, including long-sleeved cover jacket.			
2. Selects the correct size and thickness wrapping material.	0 1 2 3		
3. Places process indicator with items to be wrapped.	0 1 2 3		
4. Correctly wraps the item, ensuring the wrapper is smooth with no gaps.	0 1 2 3		
5. Places outer process monitor tape and labels the item.	0 1 2 3		
6. Places run sticker on wrapper.	0 1 2 3		
Total			

SCORE

18	Proficient
12–17	Partially Proficient—Needs Remediation
Below 12	Unsatisfactory—Not Passing

Comments:

_____

_____

_____

_____

Student Signature: _____

Instructor Signature: _____

Terminal Disinfection of OR

Student's Name: _____ Date: _____

Task: Student will demonstrate the correct technique for terminal disinfection of the OR.

Equipment and Supplies:

- Disinfectants
- Mop and bucket
- Wet vacuum
- **Cleaning supplies**

Evaluation Directions: Place the appropriate number indicating the student's proficiency for each element using the following rating scale:

3—PROFICIENT. Can perform the task. Meets minimum entry level.

2—PARTIALLY PROFICIENT. Can perform most of the task. Needs assistance. Needs constant supervision.

1—LIMITED. Can do a limited amount of the task. Must be told what to do. Needs extremely close supervision.

0—UNSATISFACTORY. Cannot perform the task. Lacks knowledge, skills, and critical thinking skills while performing the task.

Skills	Grade	Self-Assessment	Instructor Initial
Student cleans and disinfects all exposed surfaces, including the following:			
1. OR table, including mattress, extensions, and safety straps	0 1 2 3		
2. Positioning devices	0 1 2 3		
3. Patient transfer devices	0 1 2 3		
4. OR furniture, including instrument tables, prep tables, ring stands, stools, and desks	0 1 2 3		
5. Overhead procedure lights	0 1 2 3		
6. Storage cabinets and supply carts	0 1 2 3		
7. High touch areas, doors and cabinet handles, and door edges	0 1 2 3		
8. Anesthesia work station	0 1 2 3		
9. Patient monitoring devices	0 1 2 3		
10. Computer equipment and accessories	0 1 2 3		
11. Communication equipment; phones	0 1 2 3		
12. Fixed equipment including suction regulator, suction holders, viewing monitors, ESU equipment, gas regulators	0 1 2 3		

Continued

Skills	Grade	Self-Assessment	Instructor Initial
13. Uses the correct disinfectants for environmental cleaning	0 1 2 3		
14. Disposes of cleaning solutions correctly	0 1 2 3		

SCORE

42	Proficient
28–41	Partially Proficient—Needs Remediation
Below 28	Unsatisfactory—Not Passing

Comments:

_____

_____

_____

_____

Student Signature: _____

Instructor Signature: _____

Operate Gas Plasma Sterilizer

Student's Name: _____ Date: _____

Task: Student will demonstrate the correct technique for sterilizing items in a hydrogen peroxide sterilizer.

Equipment and Supplies:

- Assembles specific sterilization trays, mats, and wrapping materials approved for plasma gas sterilization
- Biological indicator and processor
- Process indicators specific to gas plasma sterilization

Evaluation Directions: Place the appropriate number indicating the student's proficiency for each element using the following rating scale:

3—PROFICIENT. Can perform the task. Meets minimum entry level.

2—PARTIALLY PROFICIENT. Can perform most of the task. Needs assistance. Needs constant supervision.

1—LIMITED. Can do a limited amount of the task. Must be told what to do. Needs extremely close supervision.

0—UNSATISFACTORY. Cannot perform the task. Lacks knowledge, skills, and critical thinking skills while performing the task.

Skills	Grade	Self-Assessment	Instructor Initial
1. Student gathers all supplies required for gas plasma sterilization selecting those specifically indicated for the sterilizer; ensures that instruments have been completely dried.	0 1 2 3		
2. Ensures that packages for sterilization have been prepared correctly using wrapping materials and chemical monitors designed only for gas plasma sterilization.	0 1 2 3		
3. Places the biological indicator correctly inside the sterilizer.	0 1 2 3		
4. Loads the sterilizer correctly according the manufacturer's IFU.	0 1 2 3		
5. Correctly enters data for the specific load.	0 1 2 3		
6. Obtains hydrogen peroxide cassette and checks for integrity.	0 1 2 3		
7. Positions the cassette correctly and inserts.	0 1 2 3		
8. Closes the system door.	0 1 2 3		
9. Selects the correct cycle and activates the sterilizer.	0 1 2 3		
10. When cycle is complete, retrieves the cycle printout and places it in sterilization log according to facility policy.	0 1 2 3		
11. Processes the biological indicator according to processor IFU; documents the result.	0 1 2 3		
Total			

SCORE

33	Proficient
22–32	Partially Proficient—Needs Remediation
Below 22	Unsatisfactory—Not Passing

Comments:

_____

_____

_____

_____

Student Signature: _____

Instructor Signature: _____

Operate Steam Sterilizer

Student's Name: _____ Date: _____

Task: Student will demonstrate the correct technique for loading and operating a steam sterilizer.

Equipment and Supplies:

- Wrapped items for sterilization
- Sterilization log
- Steam sterilizer

Evaluation Directions: Place the appropriate number indicating the student's proficiency for each element using the following rating scale:

3—PROFICIENT. Can perform the task. Meets minimum entry level.

2—PARTIALLY PROFICIENT. Can perform most of the task. Needs assistance. Needs constant supervision.

1—LIMITED. Can do a limited amount of the task. Must be told what to do. Needs extremely close supervision.

0—UNSATISFACTORY. Cannot perform the task. Lacks knowledge, skills, and critical thinking skills while performing the task.

Skills	Grade	Self-Assessment	Instructor Initial
1. Student dons correct attire, including long sleeved cover jacket.	0 1 2 3		
2. Correctly places items to be sterilized on sterilization cart; demonstrates proficiency in placing large instrument trays, basins, linen packs, and small items.	0 1 2 3		
3. Scans all items and completes documentation.	0 1 2 3		
4. Loads racks from sterilization cart correctly and secures door correctly.	0 1 2 3		
5. Selects the correct pre-programmed run cycle and activates the sterilizer.	0 1 2 3		
6. When run cycle is complete, student removes printout from sterilizer and checks each parameter; places the printout in the load documentation book according to facility protocol.	0 1 2 3		
Total			

SCORE

18	Proficient
12–17	Partially Proficient—Needs Remediation
Below 12	Unsatisfactory—Not Passing

Comments:

_____

_____

_____

_____

Student Signature: _____

Instructor Signature: _____

Operate Immediate Use (Flash) Sterilizer

Student's Name: _____ Date: _____

Task: Student will demonstrate the correct technique for processing an unwrapped instrument in immediate use (flash) steam sterilizer. Student should demonstrate nonsterile and sterile role.

Equipment and Supplies:

- Unwrapped instrument
- Sterilization tray and transfer handles
- Process indicator
- Protective eyewear
- Mask

Evaluation Directions: Place the appropriate number indicating the student's proficiency for each element using the following rating scale:

3—PROFICIENT. Can perform the task. Meets minimum entry level.

2—PARTIALLY PROFICIENT. Can perform most of the task. Needs assistance. Needs constant supervision.

1—LIMITED. Can do a limited amount of the task. Must be told what to do. Needs extremely close supervision.

0—UNSATISFACTORY. Cannot perform the task. Lacks knowledge, skills, and critical thinking skills while performing the task.

Skills	Grade	Self-Assessment	Instructor Initial
1. Student circulator dons correct attire, including long sleeved cover jacket, mask, and protective eyewear.	0 1 2 3		
2. Places instrument in sterilization tray with process monitor correctly.	0 1 2 3		
3. Secures sterilizer door correctly.	0 1 2 3		
4. Selects correct program for load and activates the sterilizer.	0 1 2 3		
5. When cycle has finished, student releases the door lock and opens the sterilizer.	0 1 2 3		
6. Student circulator dons sterile gloves and removes the instrument tray using sterile transfer forceps; transfers the tray immediately to the operating suite.	0 1 2 3		
7. Student scrub correctly removes the item from the sterilizer tray without contamination.	0 1 2 3		
Total			

SCORE

21	Proficient
14–20	Partially Proficient—Needs Remediation
Below 14	Unsatisfactory—Not Passing

Comments:

_____

_____

_____

_____

Student Signature: _____

Instructor Signature: _____

Prepare, Pack, and Transport Contaminated Supplies

Student's Name: _____ Date: _____

Task: Student will demonstrate the correct technique for "taking down" a case after surgery. This requires correct handling of supplies, solutions, linens, and their safe transport to the designated work area. It is important that the student demonstrate the procedure using a logical flow of tasks as they relate to safety, infection control, and efficiency.

Equipment and Supplies:

■ Gown and gloves
■ Prepared back table with instrument sets and other supplies in their postsurgery state
■ Ring stands and basins filled
■ Draped Mayo stand with instruments and supplies
■ Drapes and towels used and unused
■ Biohazard ("red" bags)
■ Case cart
■ Red bag linen hamper

Evaluation Directions: Place the appropriate number indicating the student's proficiency for each element using the following rating scale:

3—PROFICIENT. Can perform the task. Meets minimum entry level.

2—PARTIALLY PROFICIENT. Can perform most of the task. Needs assistance. Needs constant supervision.

1—LIMITED. Can do a limited amount of the task. Must be told what to do. Needs extremely close supervision.

0—UNSATISFACTORY. Cannot perform the task. Lacks knowledge, skills, and critical thinking skills while performing the task.

Skills	Grade	Self-Assessment	Instructor Initial
1. Student maintains sterile setup and suction until patient has left the room.	0 1 2 3		
2. Does not remove gown and gloves or protective eyewear until ready to transport equipment to decontamination area.	0 1 2 3		
3. Removes all knife blades and places them in magnetic sharps box.	0 1 2 3		
4. Places *all other* sharps in magnetic sharps box.	0 1 2 3		
5. Suctions water through suction tips.	0 1 2 3		
6. Carefully separates instruments—sharps, delicate, heavy, others in separate basins; opens all instruments fully.	0 1 2 3		
7. Places sharp instruments in a puncture resistant container.	0 1 2 3		
8. Places delicate instruments on top of heavier instruments.	0 1 2 3		
9. Places contaminated linens in linen biohazard receptacle with limited movement to prevent release of lint.	0 1 2 3		

Continued

Skills	Grade	Self-Assessment	Instructor Initial
10. Places all soft disposable items in biohazard receptacle.	0 1 2 3		
11. Suctions all fluids used to clean instruments during surgery into waste canisters.	0 1 2 3		
12. Places moist towels over instruments.	0 1 2 3		
14. Places all instruments, basins, and other nondeposable items in case cart; separates clean instruments from those that are contaminated; if case cart is not available, each tray should be placed inside biohazard bag and placed on a covered cart for transport; places a biohazard label on the cart or uses a red bag containers.	0 1 2 3		
15. Removes gown and gloves and places them in the correct receptacle.	0 1 2 3		
16. Proceeds to the decontamination area without delay.	0 1 2 3		
Total			

SCORE

48	Proficient
32–47	Partially Proficient—Needs Remediation
Below 32	Unsatisfactory—Not Passing

Comments:

_____

_____

_____

_____

Student Signature: _____

Instructor Signature: _____

Managing Scalpel Handle and Blades

Student's Name: _____ Date: _____

Task: Student will demonstrate the correct technique for mounting and removing knife blades on scalpel handles.

Equipment and Supplies:

- Knife blades #10, 11, 12, 15, 20
- Knife handles #3, 7, 9, 4
- Blunt nose needle holder
- Sharps container
- Gloves

Evaluation Directions: Place the appropriate number indicating the student's proficiency for each element using the following rating scale:

3—PROFICIENT. Can perform the task. Meets minimum entry level.

2—PARTIALLY PROFICIENT. Can perform most of the task. Needs assistance. Needs constant supervision.

1—LIMITED. Can do a limited amount of the task. Must be told what to do. Needs extremely close supervision.

0—UNSATISFACTORY. Cannot perform the task. Lacks knowledge, skills, and critical thinking skills while performing the task.

Skills	Grade	Self-Assessment	Instructor Initial
1. After donning gloves, student places all knife blades in magnetic sharps container.	0 1 2 3		
2. Using needle holder, student demonstrates correct technique for mounting and removing each blade in the correct handle.	0 1 2 3		
3. Always handles blades with needle holder.	0 1 2 3		
4. Always places blades in magnetic sharps container.	0 1 2 3		
5. Always points tip and edges of blades away from body.	0 1 2 3		
Total			

SCORE

15	Proficient
10–14	Partially Proficient—Needs Remediation
Below 10	Unsatisfactory—Not Passing

Comments:

_____

_____

_____

_____

Student Signature: _____

Instructor Signature: _____

Passing Instruments

Student's Name: _____ Date: _____

Task: Student will demonstrate the correct technique for passing types of instruments and identify common hand signals used for those instruments.

Equipment and Supplies:
- Basin instrument set and knife blades
- Gown and gloves

Evaluation Directions: Place the appropriate number indicating the student's proficiency for each element using the following rating scale:

3—PROFICIENT. Can perform the task. Meets minimum entry level.

2—PARTIALLY PROFICIENT. Can perform most of the task. Needs assistance. Needs constant supervision.

1—LIMITED. Can do a limited amount of the task. Must be told what to do. Needs extremely close supervision.

0—UNSATISFACTORY. Cannot perform the task. Lacks knowledge, skills, and critical thinking skills while performing the task.

Skills	Grade	Self-Assessment	Instructor Initial
1. Student correctly demonstrates the hand signal for knife or scalpel.	0 1 2 3		
2. Correctly demonstrates how to pass the scalpel safely.	0 1 2 3		
3. Correctly demonstrates the hand signal for thumb forceps.	0 1 2 3		
4. Correctly demonstrates how to pass tissue forceps.	0 1 2 3		
5. Correctly demonstrates the hand signal for a hemostatic clamp.	0 1 2 3		
6. Correctly demonstrates how to pass a hemostat.	0 1 2 3		
7. Correctly demonstrates hand signal for scissors.	0 1 2 3		
8. Correctly demonstrates how to pass scissors.	0 1 2 3		
9. Correctly demonstrates hand signal for suture.	0 1 2 3		
10. Correctly demonstrates how to pass loaded needle holder to right-handed and left-handed surgeon.	0 1 2 3		
11. Correctly demonstrates how to pass a retractor.	0 1 2 3		
12. Correctly demonstrates how to pass micro instruments.	0 1 2 3		
Total			

SCORE

36	Proficient
24–35	Partially Proficient—Needs Remediation
Below 24	Unsatisfactory—Not Passing

Comments:

_____

_____

_____

_____

Student Signature: _____

Instructor Signature: _____

Instrument Assembly: Balfour Retractor

Student's Name: _____ Date: _____

Task: Student should show proficiency in assembly and disassembly of Balfour retractor.

Evaluation Directions: Place the appropriate number indicating the student's proficiency for each element using the following rating scale:

3—PROFICIENT. Can perform the task. Meets minimum entry level.

2—PARTIALLY PROFICIENT. Can perform most of the task. Needs assistance. Needs constant supervision.

1—LIMITED. Can do a limited amount of the task. Must be told what to do. Needs extremely close supervision.

0—UNSATISFACTORY. Cannot perform the task. Lacks knowledge, skills and critical thinking while skills performing the task.

Skills	Grade	Self-Assessment	Instructor Initial
1. Able to assemble and disassemble Balfour retractor and accessories.	0 1 2 3		

SCORE

3	Proficient
2	Partially Proficient—Needs Remediation
Less than 2	Limited/Unsatisfactory—Not Passing

Comments:

_____

_____

_____

_____

Student Signature: _____

Instructor Signature: _____

Instrument Assembly: Kerrison Ronguer

Student's Name: _____ Date: _____

Task: Student should show proficiency in disassembly and assembly of Kerrison Ronguer.

Evaluation Directions: Place the appropriate number indicating the student's proficiency for each element using the following rating scale:

3—PROFICIENT. Can perform the task. Meets minimum entry level.

2—PARTIALLY PROFICIENT. Can perform most of the task. Needs assistance. Needs constant supervision.

1—LIMITED. Can do a limited amount of the task. Must be told what to do. Needs extremely close supervision.

0—UNSATISFACTORY. Cannot perform the task. Lacks knowledge, skills and critical thinking while skills performing the task.

Skills	Grade	Self-Assessment	Instructor Initial
1. Student should show proficiency in disassembly and assembly of Kerrison Ronguer.	0 1 2 3		

SCORE

3	Proficient
2	Partially Proficient—Needs Remediation
Less than 2	Limited/Unsatisfactory—Not Passing

Comments:

_____

_____

_____

_____

Student Signature: _____

Instructor Signature: _____

Instrument Assembly: Bookwalter/Omni Retractor

Student's Name: _____ Date: _____

Task: Student should show proficiency in assembly and disassembly of Bookwalter or Omni retractor.

Evaluation Directions: Place the appropriate number indicating the student's proficiency for each element using the following rating scale:

3—PROFICIENT. Can perform the task. Meets minimum entry level.

2—PARTIALLY PROFICIENT. Can perform most of the task. Needs assistance. Needs constant supervision.

1—LIMITED. Can do a limited amount of the task. Must be told what to do. Needs extremely close supervision.

0—UNSATISFACTORY. Cannot perform the task. Lacks knowledge, skills and critical thinking while skills performing the task.

Skills	Grade	Self-Assessment	Instructor Initial
1. Able to assemble and dissassemble Omni or Bookwalter retractor including accessories.	0 1 2 3		

SCORE

3	Proficient
2	Partially Proficient—Needs Remediation
Less than 2	Limited/Unsatisfactory—Not Passing

Comments:

_____

_____

_____

_____

Student Signature: _____

Instructor Signature: _____

Instrument Assembly: O'Sullivan O'Conner Retractor

Student's Name: _____ Date: _____

Task: Student should show proficiency in assembly and disassembly of O'Sullivan O'Conner retractor.

Evaluation Directions: Place the appropriate number indicating the student's proficiency for each element using the following rating scale:

3—PROFICIENT. Can perform the task. Meets minimum entry level.

2—PARTIALLY PROFICIENT. Can perform most of the task. Needs assistance. Needs constant supervision.

1—LIMITED. Can do a limited amount of the task. Must be told what to do. Needs extremely close supervision.

0—UNSATISFACTORY. Cannot perform the task. Lacks knowledge, skills and critical thinking while skills performing the task.

Skills	Grade	Self-Assessment	Instructor Initial
1. Able to assemble and disassemble O'Sullivan O'Conner retractor including attachments.	0 1 2 3		

SCORE

3	Proficient
2	Partially Proficient—Needs Remediation
Less than 2	Limited/Unsatisfactory—Not Passing

Comments:

_____

_____

_____

_____

Student Signature: _____

Instructor Signature: _____

Receiving Medications on Sterile Field

Student's Name: _____ Date: _____

Task: Student will demonstrate the correct technique for receiving liquid medications on the sterile field using a syringe and needle.

Equipment and Supplies:

- Medication vial
- 10 and 30 mL syringes
- Blunt tip needle
- Medicine cup/basin
- Medicine labels and waterproof marker with fine point

Evaluation Directions: Place the appropriate number indicating the student's proficiency for each element using the following rating scale:

3—PROFICIENT. Can perform the task. Meets minimum entry level.

2—PARTIALLY PROFICIENT. Can perform most of the task. Needs assistance. Needs constant supervision.

1—LIMITED. Can do a limited amount of the task. Must be told what to do. Needs extremely close supervision.

0—UNSATISFACTORY. Cannot perform the task. Lacks knowledge, skills, and critical thinking skills while performing the task.

Skills	Grade	Self-Assessment	Instructor Initial
1. Student is able to describe the rationale for the techniques used in the procedure.	0 1 2 3		
2. Student correctly prepares syringe and blunt needle.	0 1 2 3		
3. Student correctly follows drug protocol for visual assessment, identification and verbalization of drug name, strength, and maximum dose with circulator.	0 1 2 3		
4. After removing the safety cap aseptically, the circulator holds the vial for the student to receive the medication. Student inserts blunt needle into the vial stopper and withdraws the medication.	0 1 2 3		
5. Student and circulator again perform the correct protocol for identification and verbalization of the drug name, strength, and maximum dose.	0 1 2 3		
6. Student correctly injects the medication into a medication cup or basin without causing it to foam.	0 1 2 3		
7. Student immediately labels the medication container and syringe correctly.	0 1 2 3		
Total			

SCORE

21	Proficient
14–20	Partially Proficient—Needs Remediation
Below 14	Unsatisfactory—Not Passing

Comments:

_____

_____

_____

_____

Student Signature: _____

Instructor Signature: _____

Glass Ampule and Filter Needle

Student's Name: _____ Date: _____

Task: Student should demonstrate how to safely open a glass ampule and draw up liquid using a filter needle. The student should also demonstrate the safe management of glass chards and needle.

Evaluation Directions: Place the appropriate number indicating the student's proficiency for each element using the following rating scale:

3—PROFICIENT. Can perform the task. Meets minimum entry level.

2—PARTIALLY PROFICIENT. Can perform most of the task. Needs assistance. Needs constant supervision.

1—LIMITED. Can do a limited amount of the task. Must be told what to do. Needs extremely close supervision.

0—UNSATISFACTORY. Cannot perform the task. Lacks knowledge, skills and critical thinking while skills performing the task.

Skills	Grade	Self-Assessment	Instructor Initial
1. Demonstrates how to safely open a glass ampule on the sterile field.	0 1 2 3		
2. Demonstrates how to draw up liquid from the glass vial safely using a filter needle.	0 1 2 3		
3. Manages glass chards and empty ampule.	0 1 2 3		
4. Exchanges filter needle for standard needle; manages the filter needle safely	0 1 2 3		

SCORE

12	Proficient
8–11	Partially Proficient—Needs Remediation
Less than 8	Limited/Unsatisfactory—Not Passing

Comments:

_____

_____

_____

_____

Student Signature: _____

Instructor Signature: _____

Extension Tubing, Stopcock, Syringe

Student's Name: _____ Date: _____

Task: Student should demonstrate how to assemble sterile extension tubing, stopcock, syringe, and irrigation tip for injection in the wound (an olive tip irrigation needle can be used). He or she should also demonstrate how to draw up liquid and purge tubing of air, open, and close the flow valve.

Evaluation Directions: Place the appropriate number indicating the student's proficiency for each element using the following rating scale:

3—PROFICIENT. Can perform the task. Meets minimum entry level.

2—PARTIALLY PROFICIENT. Can perform most of the task. Needs assistance. Needs constant supervision.

1—LIMITED. Can do a limited amount of the task. Must be told what to do. Needs extremely close supervision.

0—UNSATISFACTORY. Cannot perform the task. Lacks knowledge, skills and critical thinking while skills performing the task.

Skills	Grade	Self-Assessment	Instructor Initial
1. Assemble sterile extension tubing, stopcock, syringe, and irrigation tip.	0 1 2 3		
2. Demonstrate closed and open positions of the flow valve.	0 1 2 3		
3. Draw up fluid and purge the system of air.	0 1 2 3		

SCORE

9	Proficient
6–8	Partially Proficient—Needs Remediation
Less than 6	Limited/Unsatisfactory—Not Passing

Comments:

_____

_____

_____

_____

Student Signature: _____

Instructor Signature: _____

Computer Basics

Student's Name: _____ Date: _____

Task: Student should demonstrate basic computer skills needed to enter data on a hospital record; perform basic research on the internet; open, create, and save a document; create an email.

Evaluation Directions: Place the appropriate number indicating the student's proficiency for each element using the following rating scale:

3—PROFICIENT. Can perform the task. Meets minimum entry level.

2—PARTIALLY PROFICIENT. Can perform most of the task. Needs assistance. Needs constant supervision.

1—LIMITED. Can do a limited amount of the task. Must be told what to do. Needs extremely close supervision.

0—UNSATISFACTORY. Cannot perform the task. Lacks knowledge, skills and critical thinking while skills performing the task.

Skills	Grade	Self-Assessment	Instructor Initial
1. Login; Logout	0 1 2 3		
2. Select program and open; close program	0 1 2 3		
3. Enter data on a form using arrow keys to position curser	0 1 2 3		
4. Save data on a form	0 1 2 3		
5. Create an email	0 1 2 3		
6. Open, create, and save a document in Word or Excell	0 1 2 3		
7. Perform basic research using the internet	0 1 2 3		

SCORE

21	Proficient
14–20	Partially Proficient—Needs Remediation
Less than 14	Limited/Unsatisfactory—Not Passing

Comments:

_____

_____

_____

_____

Student Signature: _____

Instructor Signature: _____

Assembly and Application of Patient Return Electrode (PRE)

Student's Name: _____ Date: _____

Task: Student will demonstrate the correct technique for applying PRE to patient's skin and connecting power cable.

Equipment and Supplies:

- Patient return electrode
- PRE power cable

Evaluation Directions: Place the appropriate number indicating the student's proficiency for each element using the following rating scale:

3—PROFICIENT. Can complete the task. Meets minimum entry level.

2—PARTIALLY PROFICIENT. Can complete most of the task. Needs assistance. Needs constant supervision.

1—LIMITED. Can complete a limited amount of the task. Must be told what to do. Needs extremely close supervision.

0—UNSATISFACTORY. Cannot perform the task. Lacks knowledge, skills, and critical thinking skills while performing the task.

Skills	Grade	Self-Assessment	Instructor Initial
1. Student is able to explain the purpose of the PRE and describe the path of electricity from the ESU control unit through the active electrode and back through the PRE.	0 1 2 3		
2. Student demonstrates understanding of the risks associated with faulty circuitry through the PRE.	0 1 2 3		
3. Assembles supplies—PRE in *sealed* package and power cable. Inspects power cable for integrity.	0 1 2 3		
4. Selects an appropriate site for PRE placement according to incision site and patient build. Ensures area is dry, clean, and free of hair.	0 1 2 3		
5. Checks expiry date on PRE package.	0 1 2 3		
6. Opens and assesses the PRE for ample gel.	0 1 2 3		
7. Places pad securely on the patient's skin.	0 1 2 3		
8. Connects power cable securely to pad.	0 1 2 3		
9. Is able to describe the skin site after removing the pad.	0 1 2 3		
10. Correctly documents condition of PRE site and location in the patient chart.	0 1 2 3		
Total			

SCORE

30	Proficient
20—29	Partially Proficient—Needs Remediation
Below 20	Unsatisfactory—Not Passing

Comments:

_____

_____

_____

_____

Student Signature: _____

Instructor Signature: _____

Electrosurgery Unit (ESU) Generator and its Controls

Student's Name: _____ Date: _____

Task: Student should demonstrate how to connect the patient return electrode cable to the generator. He or she should also identify the basic panel controls and what each one does. Electrosurgical units across manufacturers vary in their complexity and ability to perform multiple types of energy. Students should understand the basic functions common to all ESUs.

Evaluation Directions: Place the appropriate number indicating the student's proficiency for each element using the following rating scale:

3—PROFICIENT. Can perform the task. Meets minimum entry level.

2—PARTIALLY PROFICIENT. Can perform most of the task. Needs assistance. Needs constant supervision.

1—LIMITED. Can do a limited amount of the task. Must be told what to do. Needs extremely close supervision.

0—UNSATISFACTORY. Cannot perform the task. Lacks knowledge, skills and critical thinking while skills performing the task.

Skills	Grade	Self-Assessment	Instructor Initial
1. Demonstrates the cable connections between the foot switching monopolar instrument to the ESU generator receptacle.	0 1 2 3		
2. Demonstrates the cable connections between the hand switching monopolar cable and the ESU generator receptacle.	0 1 2 3		
3. Demonstrates the cable connection between the foot switching bipolar instruments to the bipolar ESU receptacle.	0 1 2 3		
4. Demonstrates the cable connection between the foot switching bipolar instruments to the bipolar ESU receptacle.	0 1 2 3		
5. Demonstrates the cable connection between the monopolar patient return electrode (PRE) and the ESU generator PRE receptacle.	0 1 2 3		
6. Identifies the front panel bipolar controls including power settings and mode settings.	0 1 2 3		
7. Identifies the front panel monopolar settings including coagulation and cut settings.	0 1 2 3		
8. Identifies the ESU generator power switch.	0 1 2 3		
9. Demonstrates the monopolar footswitch receptacle.	0 1 2 3		
10. Demonstrates the bipolar footswitch receptacle.	0 1 2 3		
11. Demonstrates the volume control for alarms and modes.	0 1 2 3		

Skills	Grade	Self-Assessment	Instructor Initial
12. Demonstrates the ESU power entry cable receptacle and mains receptacle.			

SCORE

36   Proficient

24–35   Partially Proficient—Needs Remediation

Less than 24   Limited/Unsatisfactory—Not Passing

Comments:

_____

_____

_____

_____

Student Signature: _____

Instructor Signature: _____

Prepare Gurney (Stretcher) and Demonstrate Use

Student's Name: _____ Date: _____

Task: Student will demonstrate the necessary preparation of a gurney for patient transport, gurney operations, and safe transport of the patient by gurney. A second student may act as a patient during demonstration of safe transport. Correctly transferring the patient from the bed to the gurney is a separate exercise. Note that if a ramp is not available, the student should describe this maneuver.

Equipment and Supplies:

■ Gurney
■ Sheets, blanket, pillow

Evaluation Directions: Place the appropriate number indicating the student's proficiency for each element using the following rating scale:

3—PROFICIENT. Can complete the task. Meets minimum entry level.

2—PARTIALLY PROFICIENT. Can complete most of the task. Needs assistance. Needs constant supervision.

1—LIMITED. Can complete a limited amount of the task. Must be told what to do. Needs extremely close supervision.

0—UNSATISFACTORY. Cannot perform the task. Lacks knowledge, skills, and critical thinking skills while performing the task.

Skills	Grade	Self-Assessment	Instructor Initial
Gurney Preparation			
1. Student correctly identifies gurney steering mechanism—brake, neutral position, forward steer.	0 1 2 3		
2. Demonstrates correct use of side rails.	0 1 2 3		
3. Demonstrates correct placement of safety strap.			
4. Demonstrates how to raise the head of gurney.	0 1 2 3		
5. Demonstrates Trendelenberg and reverse Trendelenberg tilt.	0 1 2 3		
6. Demonstrates use of IV hanger in correct position and locked.	0 1 2 3		
7. Identifies location of oxygen tank cradle.	0 1 2 3		
8. Demonstrates how to remove and replace back board.	0 1 2 3		
9. Identifies load limit (carrying capacity) label on gurney.	0 1 2 3		
Safe Patient Transport			
1. Ensures that mattress is smoothly covered with clean linen and that a blanket and pillow are on board.	0 1 2 3		
2. Correctly positions the safety strap and raises side rails.	0 1 2 3		

Skills	Grade	Self-Assessment	Instructor Initial
With patient on board, student demonstrates the following:			
1. Raising gurney to his or her hip height.	0 1 2 3		
2. Straight steering.	0 1 2 3		
3. Turning corners using wall-mounted mirrors.	0 1 2 3		
4. Tight maneuver (e.g., bringing gurney into small patient care area).	0 1 2 3		
5. Stop and brake.	0 1 2 3		
6. Travel through automatic doorways.	0 1 2 3		
7. Travel through a doorway that must be secured open.	0 1 2 3		
8. Stopping, entering, and exiting elevator. Demonstrates brake on while in elevator.	0 1 2 3		
9. Traveling up and down a ramp.	0 1 2 3		
10. Provides reassurance to patient. Provides for patient comfort (e.g., asking if patient would like another blanket or head of bed raised).	0 1 2 3		
11. Reminds patient to keep elbows and hands inside.	0 1 2 3		
12. Alerts patient to any uneven floor surfaces such as ridge at·elevator opening.	0 1 2 3		
Total			

SCORE

69	Proficient
46—68	Partially Proficient—Needs Remediation
Below 46	Unsatisfactory—Not Passing

Comments:

_____

_____

_____

_____

Student Signature: _____

Instructor Signature: _____

Transport Patient by Wheelchair

Student's Name: _____ Date: _____

Task: Student will demonstrate the correct technique required to safely transport a patient by wheelchair.

Equipment and Supplies:

■ Wheelchair
■ Blanket

Evaluation Directions: Place the appropriate number indicating the student's proficiency for each element using the following rating scale:

3—PROFICIENT. Can complete the task. Meets minimum entry level.

2—PARTIALLY PROFICIENT. Can complete most of the task. Needs assistance. Needs constant supervision.

1—LIMITED. Can complete a limited amount of the task. Must be told what to do. Needs extremely close supervision.

0—UNSATISFACTORY. Cannot perform the task. Lacks knowledge, skills, and critical thinking skills while performing the task.

Skills	Grade	Self-Assessment	Instructor Initial
Student will identify and demonstrate the use of the following wheelchair parts:			
1. Foot rests.	0 1 2 3		
2. Safety belt.	0 1 2 3		
3. Wheel brakes.	0 1 2 3		
4. Arm rest locks.	0 1 2 3		
5. IV hanger.	0 1 2 3		
6. Oxygen tank cradle.	0 1 2 3		
7. Documents pouch.	0 1 2 3		
The student should demonstrate safe transport of the patient in a wheelchair:			
1. Secures the patient in the wheelchair correctly with brakes set.	0 1 2 3		
2. Provides the patient with a blanket.	0 1 2 3		
3. Secures the patient's documents in the document rack.	0 1 2 3		
4. Demonstrates straight ahead travel.	0 1 2 3		
5. Demonstrates travel around corners using wall-mounted mirror.	0 1 2 3		
6. Enters, stops, and exits an elevator.	0 1 2 3		

Skills	Grade	Self-Assessment	Instructor Initial
7. Demonstrates travel up and down a ramp.	0 1 2 3		
8. Demonstrates travel through automatic doors.	0 1 2 3		
9. Demonstrates travel through closed doors that must be locked in open position.	0 1 2 3		
Total			

SCORE

48	Proficient
32—47	Partially Proficient—Needs Remediation
Below 32	Unsatisfactory—Not Passing

Comments:

_____

_____

_____

_____

Student Signature: _____

Instructor Signature: _____

Assisted Lateral Transfer Using Transfer Device

Student's Name: _____ Date: _____

Task: Student will demonstrate the correct technique for assisting in a lateral transfer of the patient using a transfer device. At least four people are needed to safely perform the transfer. The student should be positioned at the patient's torso to perform the log roll. The anesthesia provider manages the patient's head. One person manages the legs and feet. Large patients require additional team members at the shoulder and torso.

Equipment and Supplies:

■ Transfer device (roller or board)
■ Gurney
■ Operating table

Evaluation Directions: Place the appropriate number indicating the student's proficiency for each element using the following rating scale:

3—PROFICIENT. Can complete the task. Meets minimum entry level.

2—PARTIALLY PROFICIENT. Can complete most of the task. Needs assistance. Needs constant supervision.

1—LIMITED. Can complete a limited amount of the task. Must be told what to do. Needs extremely close supervision.

0—UNSATISFACTORY. Cannot perform the task. Lacks knowledge, skills, and critical thinking skills while performing the task.

Skills	Grade	Self-Assessment	Instructor Initial
1. Student is able to describe the safety precautions required to perform the skill.	0 1 2 3		
2. Student demonstrates strong teamwork during the maneuver.	0 1 2 3		
3. Student performs the task safely, protecting both the patient and his or her own body from injury.	0 1 2 3		
4. Ensures that gurney is aligned with OR table without gapping; sets brake lock.	0 1 2 3		
5. Ensures that all tubes, catheters, and lines are freed up and transferred before starting the maneuver.	0 1 2 3		
6. Follows the team leader's directions during the maneuver.	0 1 2 3		
7. Maintains the patient's spine in neutral position throughout the maneuver.	0 1 2 3		
8. Positions hands correctly during the maneuver.	0 1 2 3		
9. Rolls the patient to lateral position, maintaining contact with the patient during the maneuver.	0 1 2 3		
10. With transfer device in place, lowers the patient back to supine position on the device. Performs this stage in unison with the other team members as directed by one person.	0 1 2 3		

Skills	Grade	Self-Assessment	Instructor Initial
11. Protects patient as needed as the patient and transfer board is shifted to the gurney.	0 1 2 3		
12. Patient is log rolled to lateral position away from the transfer device. Student removes the transfer board.	0 1 2 3		
13. Ensures that side rails are raised immediately after completing the transfer.	0 1 2 3		
Total			

SCORE

39   Proficient

26—38   Partially Proficient—Needs Remediation

Below 26   Unsatisfactory—Not Passing

Comments:

_____

_____

_____

_____

Student Signature: _____

Instructor Signature: _____

Lateral Transfer Mobile Patient

Student's Name: _____ Date: _____

Task: Student will demonstrate the correct technique for assisting the patient in a lateral transfer from bed to gurney or from gurney to OR table. A transfer device is not required. At least two people are required for this skill.

Equipment and Supplies:

- Bed
- Gurney

Evaluation Directions: Place the appropriate number indicating the student's proficiency for each element using the following rating scale:

3—PROFICIENT. Can complete the task. Meets minimum entry level.

2—PARTIALLY PROFICIENT. Can complete most of the task. Needs assistance. Needs constant supervision.

1—LIMITED. Can complete a limited amount of the task. Must be told what to do. Needs extremely close supervision.

0—UNSATISFACTORY. Cannot perform the task. Lacks knowledge, skills, and critical thinking skills while performing the task.

Skills	Grade	Self-Assessment	Instructor Initial
1. Student is able to describe the safety precautions required in this skill.	0 1 2 3		
2. Student positions himself or herself at the side of the OR table to receive the patient. Another team member is positioned at the gurney side to assist.	0 1 2 3		
3. Ensures that gurney is aligned with OR table and sets brake.	0 1 2 3		
4. Frees up tubes, catheters, and lines; transfers IV and drainage containers to OR table side.	0 1 2 3		
5. Cautions patient to move slowly from the gurney onto the OR table.	0 1 2 3		
6. Guides the patient verbally, providing encouragement and direction as needed.	0 1 2 3		
7. Applies safety strap as soon as the patient has completed the move.	0 1 2 3		
8. Provides blanket to patient.	0 1 2 3		
9. Ensures that patient is not left alone.	0 1 2 3		
Total			

SCORE

27	Proficient
18–26	Partially Proficient—Needs Remediation
Below 18	Unsatisfactory—Not Passing

Comments:

_____

_____

_____

_____

Student Signature: _____

Instructor Signature: _____

Supine Position

Student's Name: _____ Date: _____

Task: Student will demonstrate the correct technique for placing the patient in supine position. The student should review Chapter 18 for details of safety precautions and correct use of positioning accessories; these should be demonstrated during the evaluation. Students should work in groups of four.

Equipment and Supplies:

- OR table with clean linen and safety strap
- Positioning devices

Evaluation Directions: Place the appropriate number indicating the student's proficiency for each element using the following rating scale:

3—PROFICIENT. Can complete the task. Meets minimum entry level.

2—PARTIALLY PROFICIENT. Can complete most of the task. Needs assistance. Needs constant supervision.

1—LIMITED. Can complete a limited amount of the task. Must be told what to do. Needs extremely close supervision.

0—UNSATISFACTORY. Cannot perform the task. Lacks knowledge, skills, and critical thinking skills while performing the task.

Skills	Grade	Self-Assessment	Instructor Initial
1. Student demonstrates the correlation between specific pressure points and nerve/blood vessel injury.	0 1 2 3		
2. Secures safety strap correctly.	0 1 2 3		
3. Maintains the patient's cervical spine in neutral position during positioning.	0 1 2 3		
4. Correctly positions and secures patient's arms on armboards, protecting pressure points and brachial plexus.	0 1 2 3		
5. Demonstrates correct position and use of draw sheet to secure patient's arms at sides.	0 1 2 3		
6. Protects cranial pressure point correctly.	0 1 2 3		
7. Protects sacrum correctly.	0 1 2 3		
8. For male patient, correctly positions genitalia.	0 1 2 3		
9. Protects popliteal spaces correctly.	0 1 2 3		
10. Protects Achilles tendons, ankles, and heels using correct techniques.	0 1 2 3		
Total			

SCORE

30	Proficient
20–29	Partially Proficient—Needs Remediation
Below 20	Unsatisfactory—Not Passing

Comments:

_____

_____

_____

_____

Student Signature: _____

Instructor Signature: _____

Lateral Position

Student's Name: _____ Date: _____

Task: Student will demonstrate the correct technique required to place the patient in lateral decubitus (lateral) position. Students may work in teams of four, with each student being graded on his or her specific role in the procedure. Student should review Chapter 18 for each safety point of this skill. The anesthesia provider will maintain control of the patient's head and neck in order to protect the airway.

Equipment and Supplies:

- OR table with linens and safety strap
- Table accessories
- Positioning aids

Evaluation Directions: Place the appropriate number indicating the student's proficiency for each element using the following rating scale:

3—PROFICIENT. Can perform the task. Meets minimum entry level.

2—PARTIALLY PROFICIENT. Can perform most of the task. Needs assistance. Needs constant supervision.

1—LIMITED. Can do a limited amount of the task. Must be told what to do. Needs extremely close supervision.

0—UNSATISFACTORY. Cannot perform the task. Lacks knowledge, skills, and critical thinking skills while performing the task.

Skills	Grade	Self-Assessment	Instructor Initial
1. Student demonstrates the correlation between specific pressure points and nerve/blood vessel injury.	0 1 2 3		
2. Prepares and assembles all required padding and table accessories.	0 1 2 3		
3. Positions vac pac correctly on OR table.	0 1 2 3		
4. Student participates in moving patient to operating table safely.	0 1 2 3		
5. Applies safety strap and places arms on arm boards correctly and securely.	0 1 2 3		
6. Following induction and intubation, ensures that patient's eyes are taped for protection.	0 1 2 3		
7. Team log rolls the patient to lateral position, centered on the OR table.	0 1 2 3		
8. Maintains spine in neutral position at all times.	0 1 2 3		
9. Demonstrates coordination in moving the patient as one solid unit.	0 1 2 3		
10. Maintains normal range of motion of all affected joints during the log roll.	0 1 2 3		

Skills	Grade	Self-Assessment	Instructor Initial
11. Places head in horseshoe pad or cutaway head rest correctly to protect facial nerves, ear, and eye.	0 1 2 3		
12. Ensures that no part of the eye is in contact with the head rest.	0 1 2 3		
13. Anesthesia provider brings the downside shoulder and upper arm anteriorally.	0 1 2 3		
14. Correctly positions the axillary pad.	0 1 2 3		
15. Positions vac pac correctly to support back, flank, and abdomen, or correctly attaches lateral supports to table frame.	0 1 2 3		
16. Correctly positions the lower (dependent) arm on a foam padded rest, supponated, and secures it with tape and safety strap.	0 1 2 3		
17. Correctly places the upper (nondependent) arm in pronated position in a heavily padded arm rest or foam cradle and secures it with tape and safety strap.	0 1 2 3		
18. Correctly positions lower leg comfortably flexed and upper leg with less flexion. Correctly positions padding between the upper and lower legs.	0 1 2 3		
19. Correctly places padding under each foot.	0 1 2 3		
20. Student demonstrates good teamwork and attentiveness throughout the procedure.	0 1 2 3		
Total			

SCORE

60	Proficient
40–59	Partially Proficient—Needs Remediation
Below 40	Unsatisfactory—Not Passing

Comments:

_____

_____

_____

_____

Student Signature: _____

Instructor Signature: _____

Prone Position

Student's Name: _____ Date: _____

Task: Student will demonstrate the correct technique for placing the patient in the prone position. Students may work in groups of four. A foam chest brace (Wilson brace) may be used to elevate the thorax, or a specialized table such as an Allen spine table may be used. Students should be instructed on the mechanics, accessories, and operation of this table before proceeding to patient positioning.

Equipment and Supplies:

- Operating table with linen and safety strap
- Positioning devices and table accessories
- Gurney

Evaluation Directions: Place the appropriate number indicating the student's proficiency for each element using the following rating scale:

3—PROFICIENT. Can perform the task. Meets minimum entry level.

2—PARTIALLY PROFICIENT. Can perform most of the task. Needs assistance. Needs constant supervision.

1—LIMITED. Can do a limited amount of the task. Must be told what to do. Needs extremely close supervision.

0—UNSATISFACTORY. Cannot perform the task. Lacks knowledge, skills, and critical thinking skills while performing the task.

Skills	Grade	Self-Assessment	Instructor Initial
1. Student demonstrates knowledge about specific pressure points in prone position.	0 1 2 3		
2. Student demonstrates knowledge about respiratory clearance in prone position.	0 1 2 3		
3. Assembles equipment in the operating room.	0 1 2 3		
4. Ensures that gurney and operating table are aligned with no gaps that and gurney brakes locks are set.	0 1 2 3		
5. Correctly positions foam chest brace (if used) on operating table; if chest rolls are used, ensures they are in correct position on the table.	0 1 2 3		
6. The anesthesia provider tapes the patient's eyes following induction. When the airway is secure, student correctly participates in log roll maneuver, turning the patient to prone onto the operating table.	0 1 2 3		
7. Ensures that the patient is moved as one unit, keeping spine in neutral position at all times.	0 1 2 3		
8. Demonstrates good team work during the move.	0 1 2 3		
9. The anesthesia provider immediately checks the face and airway, ensuring that the eyes and ears clear the edges of the hollow cutout in the head support.	0 1 2 3		

Skills	Grade	Self-Assessment	Instructor Initial
10. Ensures that arms are gently rotated and extended in pronated position at an angle no greater than 90 degrees, with elbows flexed.	0 1 2 3		
11. Ensures that arm boards are padded correctly and safety straps are correctly fastened.	0 1 2 3		
12. Ensures that the shoulders and chest are adequately supported.	0 1 2 3		
13. In female patients, ensures that the breasts are positioned in the open space between the parallel chest supports.	0 1 2 3		
14. Ensures that the brachial plexus is protected from injury and there is no pressure in the axillary region.	0 1 2 3		
15. In the male patient, ensures that the genitalia are not impinged by the table or positioning devices.	0 1 2 3		
16. Ensures that the knees are adequately cushioned.	0 1 2 3		
17. Ensures support to the lower legs and ankles. Ensures that the toes do not come in contact with the table.	0 1 2 3		
18. Places safety strap over patient correctly.	0 1 2 3		
Total			

SCORE

54	Proficient
36–53	Partially Proficient—Needs Remediation
Below 36	Unsatisfactory—Not Passing

Comments:

_____

_____

_____

_____

Student Signature: _____

Instructor Signature: _____

Urinary Catheterization

Student's Name: _____ Date: _____

Task: Student will demonstrate the correct technique required to perform urinary catheterization on male and female patients. The student should demonstrate the insertion of a two-way Foley retention catheter and a straight nonretention catheter. Students may be required to show proficiency on a plastic medical model before being allowed to catheterize a patient.

Note: Commercially prepared catheter trays may contain all or some of the needed supplies. Student must demonstrate ability to aseptically prepare any supplies not included in the tray.

Equipment and Supplies:

■ Sterile catheter set with prep solution, cotton swabs, plastic forceps, 10 mL syringe, drapes, and gloves
■ Two-way Foley catheter, appropriate size
■ Straight (Robinson type) catheter, appropriate size

Evaluation Directions: Place the appropriate number indicating the student's proficiency for each element using the following rating scale:

3—PROFICIENT. Can complete the task. Meets minimum entry level.

2—PARTIALLY PROFICIENT. Can complete most of the task. Needs assistance. Needs constant supervision.

1—LIMITED. Can complete a limited amount of the task. Must be told what to do. Needs extremely close supervision.

0—UNSATISFACTORY. Cannot perform the task. Lacks knowledge, skills, and critical thinking skills while performing the task.

Skills	Grade	Self-Assessment	Instructor Initial
1. Student demonstrates knowledge of the urogenital anatomy.	0 1 2 3		
2. Explains the rationale for techniques used to maintain sterility of the dominant hand and catheter during the procedure.	0 1 2 3		
3. Checks surgeon's order for catheterization (*required*).	0 1 2 3		
4. Checks patient chart for allergies. Takes required action if patient history shows iodophor or latex allergy.	0 1 2 3		
5. Student selects the correct size sterile catheter.	0 1 2 3		
6. Performs hand antisepsis.	0 1 2 3		
7. Explains the procedure to the patient (if regional anesthesia is used during surgery).	0 1 2 3		
8. Positions patient correctly as required.	0 1 2 3		
9. Prepares sterile field for supplies using aseptic technique.	0 1 2 3		
10. Dons sterile gloves and prepares all sterile supplies correctly.	0 1 2 3		

Skills	Grade	Self-Assessment	Instructor Initial
11. If balloon is to be tested, performs this task correctly.*	0 1 2 3		
12. Drapes the urogenital area and performs skin prep correctly.	0 1 2 3		
13. Lubricates and inserts the catheter aseptically to the correct level.	0 1 2 3		
14. Attaches catheter to tubing and bag correctly.	0 1 2 3		
15. If an open system or nonretention catheter is used, directs flow of urine into collection container.	0 1 2 3		
16. Inflates balloon with correct amount of sterile water and retracts catheter to correct level.*	0 1 2 3		
17. Attaches urine collection bag to OR table. According to facility policy, secures tubing to patient's upper leg.*	0 1 2 3		
18. Gathers supplies and places them in appropriate receptacle.	0 1 2 3		
19. Documents procedure, correctly including amount of urine collected.	0 1 2 3		

* Foley catheter only.

SCORE

57	Proficient
38–56	Partially Proficient—Needs Remediation
Below 38	Unsatisfactory—Not Passing

Comments:

_____

_____

_____

_____

Student Signature: _____

Instructor Signature: _____

Skin Prep—Abdominal

Student's Name: _____ Date: _____

Task: Student will demonstrate the correct technique for the patient skin prep for an abdominal procedure. According to facility policy, the patient prep is performed using a commercially prepared alcohol-Provacrylex or iodophor solution contained within a sponge applicator. Iodophor solution intended for single patient use may also be applied with prep sponges mounted on a sponge stick.

Equipment and Supplies:

- Prep solution (single patient dose) or commercially prepared applicator
- Dry sterile prep sponges
- Sponge forceps
- Cotton swabs
- Sterile gloves
- Sterile towels

Evaluation Directions: Place the appropriate number indicating the student's proficiency for each element using the following rating scale:

3—PROFICIENT. Can perform the task. Meets minimum entry level.

2—PARTIALLY PROFICIENT. Can perform most of the task. Needs assistance. Needs constant supervision.

1—LIMITED. Can do a limited amount of the task. Must be told what to do. Needs extremely close supervision.

0—UNSATISFACTORY. Cannot perform the task. Lacks knowledge, skills, and critical thinking skills while performing the task.

Skills	Grade	Self-Assessment	Instructor Initial
1. Student is able to discuss the purpose of the skin prep.	0 1 2 3		
2. Student checks the surgeon's order for prep solution/ tincture.	0 1 2 3		
3. If commercial prep applicator is used, student is able to describe correct technique for product.	0 1 2 3		
4. Checks patient chart for allergies. Takes appropriate action if allergy to prep solution or latex are documented in chart.	0 1 2 3		
5. Assembles prep supplies; prepares sterile field on prep table as needed. Opens sufficient number of prep dispensers.	0 1 2 3		
6. Performs hand antisepsis.	0 1 2 3		
7. Dons sterile gloves.	0 1 2 3		
8. Places sterile towels at the periphery of the prep site.	0 1 2 3		
9. Applies a small amount of prep solution to the umbilicus; cleanses the umbilicus using sterile cotton swabs, correctly discarding used swabs.	0 1 2 3		

Skills	Grade	Self-Assessment	Instructor Initial
10. Starting at cleansed umbilical area applies prep solution in concentric circles; correctly maintains concentric pattern without returning to previously treated areas.	0 1 2 3		
11. When the entire prep site has been treated, uses sterile sponges to wick pooled prep solution from the skin. Uses a fresh sponge for each area of pooled solution.	0 1 2 3		
12. Removes sterile towels correctly without touching prepped skin.	0 1 2 3		
13. Checks areas where prep solution may have seeped under the patient.	0 1 2 3		
14. Removes prep supplies and places them in appropriate receptacle.	0 1 2 3		
Total			

SCORE

42	Proficient
28–41	Partially Proficient—Needs Remediation
Below 28	Unsatisfactory—Not Passing

Comments:

_____

_____

_____

_____

Student Signature: _____

Instructor Signature: _____

Vaginal Prep

Student's Name: _____ Date: _____

Task: Student will demonstrate the correct technique for performing a vaginal prep.

Equipment and Supplies:
- Prep kit
- Sterile sponges
- Sponge forceps
- Prep solution
- Sterile towels
- Sterile plastic under buttocks drape

Evaluation Directions: Place the appropriate number indicating the student's proficiency for each element using the following rating scale:

3—PROFICIENT. Can perform the task. Meets minimum entry level.

2—PARTIALLY PROFICIENT. Can perform most of the task. Needs assistance. Needs constant supervision.

1—LIMITED. Can do a limited amount of the task. Must be told what to do. Needs extremely close supervision.

0—UNSATISFACTORY. Cannot perform the task. Lacks knowledge, skills, and critical thinking skills while performing the task.

Skills	Grade	Self-Assessment	Instructor Initial
1. Is able to explain the rationale for techniques required for a perineal prep.	0 1 2 3		
2. Checks surgeon's written or verbal order for prep.	0 1 2 3		
3. Assembles needed supplies.	0 1 2 3		
4. Performs hand antisepsis.			
5. Opens prep kit on prep table, creating a small sterile field using the prep tray cover.	0 1 2 3		
6. If prep solutions are not contained in the prep kit, obtains single patient dose of prep solution.	0 1 2 3		
7. With patient in lithotomy position, places kick bucket at the foot of the table to collect prep sponges and excess fluids.	0 1 2 3		
8. Waits for anesthesia provider's approval to start the prep.	0 1 2 3		
9. Dons sterile gloves.	0 1 2 3		
10. Positions the under buttocks drape using aseptic technique, extending to the kick bucket to catch used sponges and excess prep solution.	0 1 2 3		
11. Places folded sterile towel correctly above the pubis.	0 1 2 3		

Skills	Grade	Self-Assessment	Instructor Initial
12. Begins prep across the pubis using transverse strokes to each iliac crest, extending downward over the vulva and perineum. Uses correct aseptic technique. Discards sponge in kick bucket.	0 1 2 3		
13. Repeats pattern using correct technique with fresh sponges and solution.	0 1 2 3		
14. With fresh sponges, applies solution correctly to inner thighs from vulva outwards; repeats with fresh sponges.	0 1 2 3		
15. Cleanses the vagina and cervix correctly using ample prep solution; uses sponges to blot the vaginal walls, removing excess prep solution.	0 1 2 3		
16. Correctly applies prep solution to the anus from top (anterior) to bottom (posterior) using one sponge for each stroke.	0 1 2 3		
17. Removes supplies and discards them in the appropriate receptacles.	0 1 2 3		
18. Documents procedure in the patient chart.	0 1 2 3		
Total			

SCORE

54	Proficient
36–53	Partially Proficient—Needs Remediation
Below 36	Unsatisfactory—Not Passing

Comments:

_____

_____

_____

_____

Student Signature: _____

Instructor Signature: _____

Leg Prep—Knee Incision

Student's Name: _____ Date: _____

Task: Student will demonstrate the correct technique for skin prep of the leg for knee surgery. The leg should be suspended in an overhead or table mounted leg holder. According to facility policy, the patient prep is performed using a commercially prepared alcohol-Provacrylex or iodophor solution contained within a sponge applicator. Iodophor solution intended for one patient use may also be applied with prep sponges mounted on a sponge stick.

Equipment and Supplies:

- Prep solution (single patient dose) or commercially prepared applicator
- Dry sterile prep sponges
- Sponge forceps
- Sterile gloves
- Sterile towels
- Nonsterile impervious bottom sheet
- Sterile adhesive plastic drape to cover tourniquet

Evaluation Directions: Place the appropriate number indicating the student's proficiency for each element using the following rating scale:

3—PROFICIENT. Can perform the task. Meets minimum entry level.

2—PARTIALLY PROFICIENT. Can perform most of the task. Needs assistance. Needs constant supervision.

1—LIMITED. Can do a limited amount of the task. Must be told what to do. Needs extremely close supervision.

0—UNSATISFACTORY. Cannot perform the task. Lacks knowledge, skills, and critical thinking skills while performing the task.

Skills	Grade	Self-Assessment	Instructor Initial
1. If commercial prep applicator is used, student is able to describe correct technique for product.	0 1 2 3		
2. Student checks the surgeon's order for prep solution/tincture.	0 1 2 3		
3. Checks patient chart for allergies. Takes appropriate action if allergy to prep solution or latex are documented in chart.	0 1 2 3		
4. Assembles prep supplies; prepares sterile field on prep table as needed.	0 1 2 3		
5. Opens a sufficient number of prep applicators (if used) or pours antiseptic solution into small basin.	0 1 2 3		
6. Performs hand antisepsis.	0 1 2 3		
7. Circulator elevates operative leg and places drip sheet over operating table to keep it dry; leg is placed in holder.	0 1 2 3		
8. Dons sterile gloves.	0 1 2 3		

Skills	Grade	Self-Assessment	Instructor Initial
9. Covers tourniquet cuff with surgical towel secured with plastic adhesive drape.	0 1 2 3		
10. Uses no touch technique with prep sponges secured in sponge forceps or uses commercial prep applicator.			
11. Student begins prep at knee and continues around the circumference and then moves to the upper and lower leg away from the knee to the tourniquet and foot.*	0 1 2 3		
12. Gathers prep supplies and discards them in appropriate receptacle.	0 1 2 3		
13. Documents prep correctly in patient chart.	0 1 2 3		

*Technique recommended by the American Board of Orthopaedic Surgery and American Academy of Orthopaedic Surgeons, 2013.

SCORE

39   Proficient

26–38   Partially Proficient—Needs Remediation

Below 26   Unsatisfactory—Not Passing

Comments:

_____

_____

_____

_____

Student Signature: _____

Instructor Signature: _____

Laparotomy Draping

Student's Name: _____ Date: _____

Task: Student will demonstrate the correct technique for draping the abdomen. Two students may work together during the procedure.

Equipment and Supplies:
- Laparotomy draping pack
- Incise drape
- Sterile towels
- Gown and gloves

Evaluation Directions: Place the appropriate number indicating the student's proficiency for each element using the following rating scale:

3—PROFICIENT. Can perform the task. Meets minimum entry level.

2—PARTIALLY PROFICIENT. Can perform most of the task. Needs assistance. Needs constant supervision.

1—LIMITED. Can do a limited amount of the task. Must be told what to do. Needs extremely close supervision.

0—UNSATISFACTORY. Cannot perform the task. Lacks knowledge, skills, and critical thinking skills while performing the task.

Skills	Grade	Self-Assessment	Instructor Initial
1. Student correctly dons gown and gloves.	0 1 2 3		
2. Assembles drapes correctly in order of use on the back table.	0 1 2 3		
3. Places plain sheet over patient's lower body at the correct level.	0 1 2 3		
4. Correctly places four towels (near side first) to square the incision site.	0 1 2 3		
5. Removes paper backing from incise drape correctly and applies it over the incision site.	0 1 2 3		
6. Correctly positions laparotomy drape over incision site and unfolds it toward the patient's feet; unfolds the upper portion of the drape and passes the upper edge to anesthesia provider.	0 1 2 3		
7. Throughout the procedure, the student cuffs his or her hands when handling drape edges.	0 1 2 3		
8. Throughout the procedure, the student unfolds the drapes using minimal movement.	0 1 2 3		
9. Student does not adjust drapes once they are in place.	0 1 2 3		
Total			

SCORE

27	Proficient
18–26	Partially Proficient—Needs Remediation
Below 18	Unsatisfactory—Not Passing

Comments:

_____

_____

_____

_____

Student Signature: _____

Instructor Signature: _____

Lithotomy Draping

Student's Name: _____ Date: _____

Task: Student will demonstrate the correct technique for draping the patient in lithotomy.

Equipment and Supplies:
- Lithotomy drape pack
- Plastic towel drape
- Sterile towels
- Gown and gloves

Evaluation Directions: Place the appropriate number indicating the student's proficiency for each element using the following rating scale:

3—PROFICIENT. Can perform the task. Meets minimum entry level.

2—PARTIALLY PROFICIENT. Can perform most of the task. Needs assistance. Needs constant supervision.

1—LIMITED. Can do a limited amount of the task. Must be told what to do. Needs extremely close supervision.

0—UNSATISFACTORY. Cannot perform the task. Lacks knowledge, skills, and critical thinking skills while performing the task.

Skills	Grade	Self-Assessment	Instructor Initial
1. After correctly donning gown and gloves, student assembles drapes on the back table in order of their use.	0 1 2 3		
2. Positions under buttocks drape correctly.	0 1 2 3		
3. Applies plastic perineal drape correctly, avoiding contamination.	0 1 2 3		
4. Places each legging correctly.	0 1 2 3		
5. Positions folded lithotomy drape and opens folds correctly.	0 1 2 3		
6. Throughout the procedure, the student handles drape edges by cuffing the hand.	0 1 2 3		
7. Throughout the procedure, the student unfolds drapes with minimal movement.	0 1 2 3		
8. Student avoids contamination of self and drapes.	0 1 2 3		
9. Student does not adjust drapes once they are in place.	0 1 2 3		
Total			

27	Proficient
18–26	Partially Proficient—Needs Remediation
Below 18	Unsatisfactory—Not Passing

Comments:

_____

_____

_____

_____

Student Signature: _____

Instructor Signature: _____

Extremity Draping

Student's Name: _____ Date: _____

Task: Student will demonstrate the correct technique for draping the leg for knee surgery. Two students may work together. There are many ways to drape the extremities. During student evaluation, he or she should demonstrate a variety of the techniques commonly used.

Equipment and Supplies:

- Gown and gloves
- Impervious half sheet
- Tube stockinet
- Coban type self-adhering bandage 4"
- Sterile towels
- Aperture drape
- Split drape
- Incise drape
- Nonpenetrating towel clamps

Evaluation Directions: Place the appropriate number indicating the student's proficiency for each element using the following rating scale:

3—PROFICIENT. Can perform the task. Meets minimum entry level.

2—PARTIALLY PROFICIENT. Can perform most of the task. Needs assistance. Needs constant supervision.

1—LIMITED. Can do a limited amount of the task. Must be told what to do. Needs extremely close supervision.

0—UNSATISFACTORY. Cannot perform the task. Lacks knowledge, skills, and critical thinking skills while performing the task.

Skills	Grade	Self-Assessment	Instructor Initial
1. After gowning and gloving correctly student correctly positions the sterile impervious drape over the nonoperative leg and operating table. (Prepped leg is suspended by nonsterile assistant.)	0 1 2 3		
2. Grasps the foot with impervious tube stockinet and correctly unfolds it toward the knee, stopping 4 to 5 inches below the patella. Secures the stockinette using a Coban bandage.	0 1 2 3		
3. Places the split drape correctly tails down 5 to 6 inches above the knee and secures the adhesive edges. Unfolds the remaining portion toward to patient's head.	0 1 2 3		
4. With the assistant holding the foot, student moves the foot and lower leg through aperture drape correctly and positions it above the knee. Correctly passes the upper portion of the drape to the anesthesia provider.	0 1 2 3		
5. Removes paper backing from incise drape and wraps it correctly around the knee, further securing the drape edges.	0 1 2 3		

Skills	Grade	Self-Assessment	Instructor Initial
6. Throughout the procedure, the student maintains aseptic technique.	0 1 2 3		
7. Opens drape folds with minimal movement.	0 1 2 3		
8. Avoids contamination throughout the procedure.	0 1 2 3		
Total			

SCORE

24	Proficient
16–23	Partially Proficient—Needs Remediation
Below 16	Unsatisfactory—Not Passing

Comments:

_____

_____

_____

_____

Student Signature: _____

Instructor Signature: _____

Opening Back Table Pack

Student's Name: _____ Date: _____

Task: Student will demonstrate the correct technique for opening a back table pack in the circulator role.

Equipment and Supplies:

■ Back table pack
■ Back table

Evaluation Directions: Place the appropriate number indicating the student's proficiency for each element using the following rating scale:

3—PROFICIENT. Can complete the task. Meets minimum entry level.

2—PARTIALLY PROFICIENT. Can complete most of the task. Needs assistance. Needs constant supervision.

1—LIMITED. Can complete a limited amount of the task. Must be told what to do. Needs extremely close supervision.

0—UNSATISFACTORY. Cannot perform the task. Lacks knowledge, skills, and critical thinking skills while performing the task.

Skills	Grade	Self-Assessment	Instructor Initial
1. Is able to explain the purpose of the task and principles of sterile technique involved in completing it.	0 1 2 3		
2. Removes the dust cover from the pack and places it in correct orientation on the back table. Inspects the outside of the pack for watermarks or holes.	0 1 2 3		
3. Places both hands under the folded cuff of the pack's cover and pulls it down and away from the pack.	0 1 2 3		
4. Shows care when pulling the cover back to avoid contaminating the inside surface of the pack cover (table drape) or the pack.	0 1 2 3		
5. Grasps only the edges of the pack cover and avoids leaning into the pack and table while working.	0 1 2 3		
6. Moves to the opposite side of the table and repeats the process on the second flap of the pack cover.	0 1 2 3		
7. Demonstrates important principle of aseptic technique by *not* adjusting the table drape once it is open.	0 1 2 3		
Total			

SCORE

21	Proficient
14–20	Partially Proficient—Needs Remediation
Below 14	Unsatisfactory—Not Passing

Comments:

_____

_____

_____

_____

Student Signature: _____

Instructor Signature: _____

Opening a Rigid Sterilization System

Student's Name: _____ Date: _____

Task: Student will demonstrate the correct technique for opening a rigid sterilization system in the nonsterile role.

Note: Rigid sterilization systems vary in design, including locking systems and filter mechanisms. Students should be tested on a system they are familiar with and have had formal instruction in.

Equipment and Supplies:
- Small table
- Sterile instrument tray system

Evaluation Directions: Place the appropriate number indicating the student's proficiency for each element using the following rating scale:

3—PROFICIENT. Can complete the task. Meets minimum entry level.

2—PARTIALLY PROFICIENT. Can complete most of the task. Needs assistance. Needs constant supervision.

1—LIMITED. Can complete a limited amount of the task. Must be told what to do. Needs extremely close supervision.

0—UNSATISFACTORY. Cannot perform the task. Lacks knowledge, skills, and critical thinking skills while performing the task.

Skills	Grade	Self-Assessment	Instructor Initial
1. Student is able to explain the principles of rigid sterilization systems including the sterile and nonsterile boundaries of the tray.	0 1 2 3		
2. Places the rigid sterilization tray in position on the table, which will enable aseptic removal of the inner tray by the scrub.	0 1 2 3		
3. Inspects the external process indicators.	0 1 2 3		
4. Inspects the tamper evident locks for integrity.	0 1 2 3		
5. Verifies the presence of a filter.	0 1 2 3		
6. Moves both handles of the container to open position, breaking the tamper evident locks.	0 1 2 3		
7. Discards all pieces of the tamper evident locks before opening the lid of the container.	0 1 2 3		
8. Fully disengages the handles and removes the lid in a continuous action up and away from the lower portion of the container.	0 1 2 3		
9. Removes the filter plate and filter. Checks the integrity of the filter. Replaces the filter plate and discards the filter in appropriate receptacle.	0 1 2 3		
10. After scrub has removed the inner instrument tray aseptically, student checks the bottom filter for integrity (if a perforated container is used).	0 1 2 3		

Skills	Grade	Self-Assessment	Instructor Initial
11. Replaces the filter plate in the bottom tray.	0 1 2 3		
12. Student and or scrub inspect the process monitor inside the instrument tray.	0 1 2 3		
Total			

SCORE

36	Proficient
24–35	Partially Proficient—Needs Remediation
Below 24	Unsatisfactory—Not Passing

Comments:

_____

_____

_____

_____

Student Signature: _____

Instructor Signature: _____

Opening Small Sterile Items

Student's Name: _____ Date: _____

Task: Student will demonstrate the correct technique to distribute small sterile items wrapped envelope style onto the sterile field (nonsterile role).

Equipment and Supplies:
- Small wrapped item(s)
- Covered back table

Evaluation Directions: Place the appropriate number indicating the student's proficiency for each element using the following rating scale:

3—PROFICIENT. Can complete the task. Meets minimum entry level.

2—PARTIALLY PROFICIENT. Can complete most of the task. Needs assistance. Needs constant supervision.

1—LIMITED. Can complete a limited amount of the task. Must be told what to do. Needs extremely close supervision.

0—UNSATISFACTORY. Cannot perform the task. Lacks knowledge, skills, and critical thinking skills while performing the task.

Skills	Grade	Self-Assessment	Instructor Initial
1. Student is able to describe the rationale for methods used in this skill.	0 1 2 3		
2. Student uses deliberate, careful movements while performing the skill.	0 1 2 3		
3. Positions the sterile package with the first flap on the far side.	0 1 2 3		
4. Checks the wrapper for watermarks, holes, and tears.	0 1 2 3		
5. Checks the process monitor on the outer wrapper.	0 1 2 3		
6. Breaks the tape securing the wrapper.	0 1 2 3		
7. Holds the package in one hand and peels the first (distant) flap back, *covering the exposed part of the hand*; secures the flap snugly in the palm of the same hand.	0 1 2 3		
8. Using the same technique, peels back the side flaps, one at a time.	0 1 2 3		
9. Pulls the nearest flap back and secures it using the same technique.	0 1 2 3		
10. Demonstrates the ability to cover all exposed parts of the hand with the wrapper flaps so that the sterile surfaces face outward.	0 1 2 3		
11. Carefully places the sterile item on the back table.	0 1 2 3		
12. Completes all parts of the skill without contamination of the item or the sterile field.	0 1 2 3		

Skills	Grade	Self-Assessment	Instructor Initial
13. Disposes of the wrapper in appropriate receptacle.	0 1 2 3		
Total			

SCORE

39	Proficient
26–38	Partially Proficient—Needs Remediation
Below 26	Unsatisfactory—Not Passing

Comments:

_____

_____

_____

_____

Student Signature: _____

Instructor Signature: _____

Distributing Sterile Items to Scrub

Student's Name: _____ Date: _____

Task: Student will demonstrate the correct technique for distributing sterile items directly to scrubbed personnel (nonsterile role demonstrated). Students may work in pairs.

Equipment and Supplies:
- Envelope wrapped surgical supplies
- Gown and gloves

Evaluation Directions: Place the appropriate number indicating the student's proficiency for each element using the following rating scale:

3—PROFICIENT. Can complete the task. Meets minimum entry level.

2—PARTIALLY PROFICIENT. Can complete most of the task. Needs assistance. Needs constant supervision.

1—LIMITED. Can complete a limited amount of the task. Must be told what to do. Needs extremely close supervision.

0—UNSATISFACTORY. Cannot perform the task. Lacks knowledge, skills, and critical thinking skills while performing the task.

Skills	Grade	Self-Assessment	Instructor Initial
1. Student is able to explain the rationale for techniques used in this skill.			
2. Student faces the scrubbed team member maintaining a safe distance.			
3. Opens the sterile package correctly opening the distant flap first followed by the side flaps and the nearest flap last.			
4. Maintains a secure hold on the sterile item and wrapper flaps until the scrubbed team member takes the item.			
5. Discards the wrapper in the appropriate receptacle.			
6. Completes all parts of the skill without contamination of the item or scrubbed team member.			
Total			

SCORE

18	Proficient
12–18	Partially Proficient—Needs Remediation
Below 12	Unsatisfactory—Not Passing

Comments:

_____

_____

_____

_____

Student Signature: _____

Instructor Signature: _____

Opening Sterile Peel Pouches

Student's Name: _____ Date: _____

Task: Student will demonstrate the correct technique for opening peel pouches in the nonsterile role. Direct distribution to a sterile team member, "flipping" technique (small commercially sealed packets), and tipping technique used with blister packs should be demonstrated.

Note: Students that are not confident in their skills using the flipping technique should practice outside of surgery to avoid contaminating supplies.

Equipment and Supplies:

■ Peel pouches containing sterile instruments or supplies
■ Team member in scrub role to assist

Note: Blister packs containing sterile items should have a semirigid transparent container sealed to a paper or transparent plastic covering. The tipping technique should be demonstrated with this type of wrapper.

Evaluation Directions: Place the appropriate number indicating the student's proficiency for each element using the following rating scale:

3—PROFICIENT. Can complete the task. Meets minimum entry level.

2—PARTIALLY PROFICIENT. Can complete most of the task. Needs assistance. Needs constant supervision.

1—LIMITED. Can complete a limited amount of the task. Must be told what to do. Needs extremely close supervision.

0—UNSATISFACTORY. Cannot perform the task. Lacks knowledge, skills, and critical thinking skills while performing the task.

Skills	Grade	Self-Assessment	Instructor Initial
1. Is able to describe the nonsterile boundaries and spaces of the peel pouch.	0 1 2 3		
2. Faces scrub personnel during demonstration. Stands a safe distance from the scrub personnel to avoid contamination.	0 1 2 3		
3. Inspects peel pouch wrapper for watermarks, holes, and tears.	0 1 2 3		
4. Inspects process monitor.	0 1 2 3		
5. Grasps the top edges of the peel pouch with one hand on each margin. Uses thumbs and first fingers to grasp edges.	0 1 2 3		
6. Peels back each side of the peel pack, everting the two sides to expose the contents of the pack.	0 1 2 3		
7. Maintains position as scrub personnel removes the contents without contaminating it on the nonsterile edges of the pouch.	0 1 2 3		

Skills	Grade	Self-Assessment	Instructor Initial
8. Demonstrates flipping technique using lightweight sterile item in peel pouch. Maintains a distance of 12 inches from the table during demonstration.	0 1 2 3		
9. Demonstrates tipping technique used with sterile blister packages. Peels back top portion of wrapper while holding the blister area firmly.	0 1 2 3		
10. Tips the item directly into the hands of the scrub personnel without allowing the item to slide over the edges of the blister area.	0 1 2 3		
11. In all demonstrations, student must dispose of the wrapper in an appropriate receptacle.	0 1 2 3		
Total			

SCORE

33   Proficient

22–32   Partially Proficient—Needs Remediation

Below 22   Unsatisfactory—Not Passing

Comments:

_____

_____

_____

_____

Student Signature: _____

Instructor Signature: _____

Pouring Sterile Solutions Aseptically

Student's Name: _____ Date: _____

Task: Student will demonstrate the correct technique for pouring sterile solutions into a basin on the sterile field, demonstrated in the nonsterile role.

Equipment and Supplies:
- Ring stand and basin
- Sealed sterile solution
- Sterile team member

Evaluation Directions: Place the appropriate number indicating the student's proficiency for each element using the following rating scale:

3—PROFICIENT. Can complete the task. Meets minimum entry level.

2—PARTIALLY PROFICIENT. Can complete most of the task. Needs assistance. Needs constant supervision.

1—LIMITED. Can complete a limited amount of the task. Must be told what to do. Needs extremely close supervision.

0—UNSATISFACTORY. Cannot perform the task. Lacks knowledge, skills, and critical thinking skills while performing the task.

Skills	Grade	Self-Assessment	Instructor Initial
1. Student is able to explain the rationale for the techniques required for the skill.	0 1 2 3		
2. Student faces sterile team member and verifies the name of the solution, strength, and expiry date. Visual and verbal verification is required of each person.	0 1 2 3		
3. Student inspects the seal over the cap for integrity, and inspects the solution itself for sediment or discoloration.	0 1 2 3		
4. Stands 12 inches from the basin used to receive the solution.	0 1 2 3		
5. Breaks the cap seal and lifts the cap upward to avoid contaminating the lip of the container.	0 1 2 3		
6. Turns the container over to distribute the solution into the basin. Distributes entire amount.	0 1 2 3		
7. Moves the container directly away from the basin while maintaining upturned position.	0 1 2 3		
8. Verifies the name and strength of the solution with the sterile team member.	0 1 2 3		
9. Places the empty container in a designated place where all other solution and medication containers will be collected during the surgery.	0 1 2 3		
Total			

SCORE

27	Proficient
18–26	Partially Proficient—Needs Remediation
Below 18	Unsatisfactory—Not Passing

Comments:

_____

_____

_____

_____

Student Signature: _____

Instructor Signature: _____

Room Preparation / Opening a Case

Student's Name: _____ Date: _____

Task: Student will demonstrate the correct technique used to prepare the operating room for surgery as part of case turnover. Skills required to open a case include general room preparation. Assessments of students' ability to prepare specific equipment are addressed as separate skill sets.

Equipment and Supplies:
- Clean operating room
- Case cart with wrapped supplies for general surgery

Evaluation Directions: Place the appropriate number indicating the student's proficiency for each element using the following rating scale:

3—PROFICIENT. Can complete the task. Meets minimum entry level.

2—PARTIALLY PROFICIENT. Can complete most of the task. Needs assistance. Needs constant supervision.

1—LIMITED. Can complete a limited amount of the task. Must be told what to do. Needs extremely close supervision.

0—UNSATISFACTORY. Cannot perform the task. Lacks knowledge, skills, and critical thinking skills while performing the task.

Skills	Grade	Self-Assessment	Instructor Initial
Room Preparation			
1. Student is methodical and systematic in preparing the room.	0 1 2 3		
2. Obtains surgeon's request card and places it with case cart.	0 1 2 3		
3. Student is correctly attired, including long-sleeved cover jacket.	0 1 2 3		
4. Checks case cart contents against surgeon request card, noting which items must be added to cart.	0 1 2 3		
5. Moves furniture that will be draped away from nonsterile surfaces, allowing at least a 12" space between nonsterile and sterile surfaces.	0 1 2 3		
6. Checks suction lines for pressure.	0 1 2 3		
7. Places clean suction canisters in their holders.	0 1 2 3		
8. Positions operating table under main lights.	0 1 2 3		
9. Covers operating table with clean linen.	0 1 2 3		
10. Ensures that safety strap is attached to operating table.	0 1 2 3		
11. Places liners in kick bucket and all waste receptacles according to type.	0 1 2 3		
12. Obtains appropriate forms for circulator duties.	0 1 2 3		

Skills	Grade	Self-Assessment	Instructor Initial
13. Assembles all needed positioning aids.	0 1 2 3		
14. Assembles needed equipment such as microscope. Student damp dusts any equipment coming from a storeroom before bringing it into the operating room.	0 1 2 3		
Opening the Case			
1. Correctly positions back table pack and opens it using aseptic technique.	0 1 2 3		
2. Places wrapped basins in ring stands and opens them using aseptic technique.	0 1 2 3		
3. Opens small items onto the back table using correct technique.	0 1 2 3		
4. Opens large instrument trays on small tables.	0 1 2 3		
5. Opens drapes, gowns, gloves, and other linens onto back table.	0 1 2 3		
6. Presents sharps and larger instruments directly to the scrub.	0 1 2 3		
7. Places all wrappers in appropriate receptacles.	0 1 2 3		
Total			

SCORE

63	Proficient
42–62	Partially Proficient—Needs Remediation
Below 42	Unsatisfactory—Not Passing

Comments:

_____

_____

_____

_____

Student Signature: _____

Instructor Signature: _____

Preparing Suction Unit

Student's Name: _____ Date: _____

Task: Student will demonstrate the correct technique for preparing a suction unit.

Equipment and Supplies:
- Suction unit including canister and vacuum gauge
- Suction tubing

Evaluation Directions: Place the appropriate number indicating the student's proficiency for each element using the following rating scale:

3—PROFICIENT. Can perform the task. Meets minimum entry level.

2—PARTIALLY PROFICIENT. Can perform most of the task. Needs assistance. Needs constant supervision.

1—LIMITED. Can do a limited amount of the task. Must be told what to do. Needs extremely close supervision.

0—UNSATISFACTORY. Cannot perform the task. Lacks knowledge, skills, and critical thinking skills while performing the task.

Skills	Grade	Self-Assessment	Instructor Initial
1. Places suction liner with fixed lid in suction canister correctly.	0 1 2 3		
2. Tests vacuum pressure correctly.	0 1 2 3		
3. Attaches suction tubing to lid correctly.	0 1 2 3		
4. Adjusts vacuum pressure.	0 1 2 3		
Total			

SCORE

12	Proficient
8–11	Partially Proficient—Needs Remediation
Below 8	Unsatisfactory—Not Passing

Comments:

_____

_____

_____

_____

Student Signature: _____

Instructor Signature: _____

Surgical Count

Student's Name: _____ Date: _____

Task: Student will demonstrate the correct technique for taking the surgical count.

Equipment and Supplies:

■ Back table set up with instrument set, sponges, suture needles, hypodermic needles
■ Gown and gloves

Evaluation Directions: Place the appropriate number indicating the student's proficiency for each element using the following rating scale:

3—PROFICIENT. Can perform the task. Meets minimum entry level.

2—PARTIALLY PROFICIENT. Can perform most of the task. Needs assistance. Needs constant supervision.

1—LIMITED. Can do a limited amount of the task. Must be told what to do. Needs extremely close supervision.

0—UNSATISFACTORY. Cannot perform the task. Lacks knowledge, skills, and critical thinking skills while performing the task.

Skills	Grade	Self-Assessment	Instructor Initial
1. Student is able to list all circumstances and tissue layers that require a count.	0 1 2 3		
2. Student counts all items systematically with circulator.	0 1 2 3		
3. When counting sponges, correctly separates each one from the others. Counts all sponges, all types; counts verbally.	0 1 2 3		
4. Counts all sharps correctly and systematically. Uses an instrument as a pointer during count.	0 1 2 3		
5. Counts all wound management supplies such as vessel loops, shods, electrode tips, vessel clips, using correct technique.	0 1 2 3		
6. Counts all instruments systematically using correct technique.	0 1 2 3		
7. Student correctly documents the count after the case.	0 1 2 3		
Total			

SCORE

21	Proficient
14–20	Partially Proficient—Needs Remediation
Below 14	Unsatisfactory—Not Passing

Comments:

_____

_____

_____

_____

Student Signature: _____

Instructor Signature: _____

Handling Suture Ties

Student's Name: _____ Date: _____

Task: Student will demonstrate the correct techniques for preparing suture ties including dividing, cutting, and straightening lengths of suture.

Equipment and Supplies:

- Gown and gloves
- Assorted suture ties 36" and 18"—chromic gut, silk, or polyester
- Suture scissors
- Small basin of water

Evaluation Directions: Place the appropriate number indicating the student's proficiency for each element using the following rating scale:

3—PROFICIENT. Can perform the task. Meets minimum entry level.

2—PARTIALLY PROFICIENT. Can perform most of the task. Needs assistance. Needs constant supervision.

1—LIMITED. Can do a limited amount of the task. Must be told what to do. Needs extremely close supervision.

0—UNSATISFACTORY. Cannot perform the task. Lacks knowledge, skills, and critical thinking skills while performing the task.

Skills	Grade	Self-Assessment	Instructor Initial
1. Student correctly demonstrates how to open chromic gut package safely, directing alcohol away from the surgical field.	0 1 2 3		
2. Correctly demonstrates rinsing and softening chromic gut.	0 1 2 3		
3. Correctly demonstrates how to straighten, divide, and cut chromic gut into ¼, ⅓, and ½ lengths.	0 1 2 3		
4. Correctly demonstrates how to straighten nylon suture with or without needle.	0 1 2 3		
5. Always maintains suture needles on a needle holder or in magnetic box.	0 1 2 3		
Total			

SCORE

15	Proficient
10–14	Partially Proficient—Needs Remediation
Below 10	Unsatisfactory—Not Passing

Comments:

_____

_____

_____

_____

Student Signature: _____

Instructor Signature: _____

Suture and Needle Management

Student's Name: _____ Date: _____

Task: Student will demonstrate the correct techniques for

- Loading and passing a swaged needle—right and left handed surgeon
- Loading free needle on needle holder, threading the needle, passing, and reloading
- Passing instrument and free hand ties
- Tagging and cutting sutures

Students may work in pairs.

Equipment and Supplies:

- Gown and gloves
- Magnetic needle box
- Assortment of swaged sutures and needle holders.
- Assortment of suture ties
- Right angle mixter and curved schnidt or similar type clamp.
- Suture scissors
- Eyed needles

Evaluation Directions: Place the appropriate number indicating the student's proficiency for each element using the following rating scale:

3—PROFICIENT. Can perform the task. Meets minimum entry level.

2—PARTIALLY PROFICIENT. Can perform most of the task. Needs assistance. Needs constant supervision.

1—LIMITED. Can do a limited amount of the task. Must be told what to do. Needs extremely close supervision.

0—UNSATISFACTORY. Cannot perform the task. Lacks knowledge, skills, and critical thinking skills while performing the task.

Skills	Grade	Self-Assessment	Instructor Initial
1. Student correctly removes suture packaging and mounts swaged needle on the appropriate size needle holder.	0 1 2 3		
2. Correctly positions and passes the NH across the table to a right-handed surgeon; ensures that the surgeon does not grasp the suture ends along with the NH.	0 1 2 3		
3. Correctly positions and passes the NH across the table to a left-handed surgeon; ensures that the surgeon does not grasp the suture ends along with the NH.	0 1 2 3		
4. Correctly performs #2 and #3 with surgeon positioned on the same side of the table as the student.	0 1 2 3		
5. Correctly mounts an eyed needle on NH; correctly threads the needle and secures the suture strand.	0 1 2 3		

Continued

Skills	Grade	Self-Assessment	Instructor Initial
6. Correctly passes the suture/needle combination to surgeon, receives empty needle and reloads; ensures that the surgeon does not grasp the suture ends along with the NH.	0 1 2 3		
7. Correctly tags a suture using the appropriate size hemostat with shods.	0 1 2 3		
8. Demonstrates the correct method for passing a free tie.	0 1 2 3		
9. Demonstrates the correct method for mounting an instrument tie, passing it to the surgeon.	0 1 2 3		
10. Demonstrates correctly how to cut sutures in the wound.	0 1 2 3		
Total			

SCORE

30	Proficient
22–29	Partially Proficient—Needs Remediation
Below 22	Unsatisfactory—Not Passing

Comments:

_____

_____

_____

_____

Student Signature: _____

Instructor Signature: _____

Management of Specimens

Student's Name: _____ Date: _____

Task: Student will demonstrate the correct technique for specimen management.

Equipment and Supplies:

- Prepared back table
- Gown and gloves
- Basic instruments including smooth tissue forceps
- Small basin set
- Specimen containers various sizes
- Specimen labels
- Small biopsy brush and container for receiving bronchial washing.
- Cup forceps used to obtain micro biopsy.
- Hypodermic needles size 18 and 21
- Marking pen, fine point
- Specimen requisition forms
- Laboratory requisition forms

Evaluation Directions: Place the appropriate number indicating the student's proficiency for each element using the following rating scale:

3—PROFICIENT. Can perform the task. Meets minimum entry level.

2—PARTIALLY PROFICIENT. Can perform most of the task. Needs assistance. Needs constant supervision.

1—LIMITED. Can do a limited amount of the task. Must be told what to do. Needs extremely close supervision.

0—UNSATISFACTORY. Cannot perform the task. Lacks knowledge, skills, and critical thinking skills while performing the task.

Skills	Grade	Self-Assessment	Instructor Initial
1. Student is able to explain the use of specimen markers (sutures, dye, or clips) and how they are used by the surgeon.	0 1 2 3		
2. Student can discuss the importance of maintaining the integrity of biopsy specimens.	0 1 2 3		
3. Student can explain the technique for maintaining forensic specimens correctly.	0 1 2 3		
4. Student correctly demonstrates how to receive a tissue specimen from the surgeon.	0 1 2 3		
5. Correctly demonstrates the use of Telfa and saline solution to keep a tissue specimen moist.	0 1 2 3		
6. Correctly demonstrates how to label a specimen on the back table.	0 1 2 3		
7. Correctly demonstrates how to transfer a tissue specimen to the circulator.	0 1 2 3		

Continued

Skills	Grade	Self-Assessment	Instructor Initial
8. Correctly verifies the specimen information with the surgeon.	0 1 2 3		
9. Correctly demonstrates how to transfer bronchial brushings to the specimen container.	0 1 2 3		
10. Correctly demonstrates how to remove microbiopsy tissue from forceps and transfer it to solution in specimen container.	0 1 2 3		
11. Demonstrates how to assist in taking microbiology specimens using a swab and transport tube; correctly prepares the specimen for aseptic transfer to pathology.	0 1 2 3		
12. Demonstrates correct method for documenting specimens for pathology.	0 1 2 3		
13. Demonstrates correct method for documenting specimens for microbiology investigation (e.g., culture).	0 1 2 3		
14. Demonstrates the correct method for safely packaging tissue specimens and requisitions for transfer to pathology.	0 1 2 3		
15. Demonstrates the correct method for maintaining specimens for frozen section.	0 1 2 3		
Total			

SCORE

45   Proficient

30–44   Partially Proficient—Needs Remediation

Below 30   Unsatisfactory—Not Passing

Comments:

_____

_____

_____

_____

Student Signature: _____

Instructor Signature: _____

Preparing Mayo Tray and Instruments

Student's Name: _____ Date: _____

Task: Student will demonstrate correct technique for draping the Mayo tray and organizing instruments. The student may demonstrate the skill using the facility's standard setup and another setup of his or her choice.

Equipment and Supplies:

- Prepared back table
- General surgery instrument set
- Gown and gloves
- Mayo stand
- Mayo drape
- Towels

Evaluation Directions: Check or circle the appropriate number to indicate the student's performance level, using the following rating scale:

3—PROFICIENT. Can perform the task. Meets minimum entry level.

2—PARTIALLY PROFICIENT. Can perform most of the task. Needs assistance. Needs constant supervision.

1—LIMITED. Can do a limited amount of the task. Must be told what to do. Needs extremely close supervision.

0—UNSATISFACTORY. Cannot perform the task. Lacks knowledge, skills, and critical thinking skills while performing the task.

Task Checklist	Grade	Self-Assessment	Instructor Initial
1. Correctly drapes the Mayo stand and tray.	0 1 2 3		
2. Place two towels and towel roll on Mayo tray.	0 1 2 3		
3. Isolates knives in one area of tray.	0 1 2 3		
4. Places scissors, tissue forceps in separate area of the tray.	0 1 2 3		
5. Places small and medium box lock instruments over towel roll.	0 1 2 3		
6. Places handheld retractors in a separate location on the tray.	0 1 2 3		
Total			

SCORE

18	Proficient
12–17	Partially Proficient—Needs Remediation
Below 12	Unsatisfactory—Not Passing

Comments:

_____

_____

_____

_____

Student Signature: _____

Instructor Signature: _____

Operating Lights

Student's Name: _____ Date: _____

Task: Student will demonstrate the operating lights controls and options.

Evaluation Directions: Place the appropriate number indicating the student's proficiency for each element using the following rating scale:

3—PROFICIENT. Can perform the task. Meets minimum entry level.

2—PARTIALLY PROFICIENT. Can perform most of the task. Needs assistance. Needs constant supervision.

1—LIMITED. Can do a limited amount of the task. Must be told what to do. Needs extremely close supervision.

0—UNSATISFACTORY. Cannot perform the task. Lacks knowledge, skills and critical thinking while skills performing the task.

Skills	Grade	Self-Assessment	Instructor Initial
1. Locate the light panel	0 1 2 3		
2. Differentiate between operating lights and room lights	0 1 2 3		
3. Activate the operating lights	0 1 2 3		
4. Adjust the brightness control	0 1 2 3		
5. Adjust the size of the beam; show overlapping and separate beams	0 1 2 3		
6. Demonstrate linear and rotating movement of lights.	0 1 2 3		
7. Demonstrate light beam angles	0 1 2 3		

SCORE

21	Proficient
14–20	Partially Proficient—Needs Remediation
Less than 14	Limited/Unsatisfactory—Not Passing

Comments:

_____

_____

_____

_____

Student Signature: _____

Instructor Signature: _____

Operating Table and Attachments

Student's Name: _____ Date: _____

Task: Student will demonstrate proficiency in moving and configuring the operating table as described below.

■ Set reverse Trendelberg
■ Flex lower articulation

Evaluation Directions: Place the appropriate number indicating the student's proficiency for each element using the following rating scale:

3—PROFICIENT. Can perform the task. Meets minimum entry level.

2—PARTIALLY PROFICIENT. Can perform most of the task. Needs assistance. Needs constant supervision.

1—LIMITED. Can do a limited amount of the task. Must be told what to do. Needs extremely close supervision.

0—UNSATISFACTORY. Cannot perform the task. Lacks knowledge, skills and critical thinking while skills performing the task.

Skills	Grade	Self-Assessment	Instructor Initial
1. Release floor lock; demonstrate how to move the table; activate the floor lock	0 1 2 3		
2. Raise and lower table height	0 1 2 3		
3. Demonstrate right and left table roll	0 1 2 3		
4. Place table in Trendelenberg position	0 1 2 3		
5. Place table in reverse Trendelenberg position	0 1 2 3		
6. Flex the lower table articulation downward as for lithotomy.	0 1 2 3		
7. Set upper, middle and lower table breaks for Fowler's position	0 1 2 3		
8. Remove and replace head section	0 1 2 3		
9. Attach and detach standard arm boards	0 1 2 3		
10. Attach and detach Allen (yellow fin) leg holders (lithotomy position)	0 1 2 3		
11. Attach and detach candy cane stirrups (lithotomy position)	0 1 2 3		
12. Attach and detach bariatric split leg extensions.	0 1 2 3		

SCORE

36	Proficient
24–35	Partially Proficient—Needs Remediation
Less than 24	Limited/Unsatisfactory—Not Passing

Comments:

_____

_____

_____

_____

Student Signature: _____

Instructor Signature: _____

Place a Pneumatic Tourniquet Cuff

Student's Name: _____ Date: _____

Task: Student will demonstrate the correct technique for positioning a pneumatic tourniquet on the arm.

Note: This procedure is normally carried out by the surgeon, his or her assistant, or the anesthesia provider according to hospital policy (as noted in Miller et al.'s *Miller's Anesthesia*, 8th ed., Saunders, 2012).

Equipment and Supplies:
- Pneumatic tourniquet device
- Tourniquet
- Webril padding

Evaluation Directions: Place the appropriate number indicating the student's proficiency for each element using the following rating scale:

3—PROFICIENT. Can perform the task. Meets minimum entry level.

2—PARTIALLY PROFICIENT. Can perform most of the task. Needs assistance. Needs constant supervision.

1—LIMITED. Can do a limited amount of the task. Must be told what to do. Needs extremely close supervision.

0—UNSATISFACTORY. Cannot perform the task. Lacks knowledge, skills, and critical thinking skills while performing the task.

Skills	Grade	Self-Assessment	Instructor Initial
1. Student demonstrates understanding of the risks involved in the use of a pneumatic tourniquet.	0 1 2 3		
2. Student obtains surgeon's written or verbal order for application of a tourniquet.	0 1 2 3		
3. Assembles supplies near the patient, including the correct size tourniquet cuff and Webril as specified by the surgeon.	0 1 2 3		
4. Ensures that the tourniquet is safe to use with no puncture sites, tears, or worn Velcro closures.	0 1 2 3		
5. Verifies the tourniquet level on the limb with surgeon.	0 1 2 3		
6. Assesses the appearance of the skin at the tourniquet site.	0 1 2 3		
7. Correctly applies adequate Webril padding to the tourniquet site with no folds or wrinkles.	0 1 2 3		
8. Positions and secures the tourniquet correctly over the Webril padding.	0 1 2 3		
Total			

SCORE

24	Proficient
16–23	Partially Proficient—Needs Remediation
Below 16	Unsatisfactory—Not Passing

Comments:

_____

_____

_____

_____

Student Signature: _____

Instructor Signature: _____

Sponge Stick and Dissection Sponges

Student's Name: _____ Date: _____

Task: Student will demonstrate the correct technique for creating a sponge stick and mounting dissection sponges.

Equipment and Supplies:

- 4 × 4 surgical sponges
- Small sponge dissectors (2 sizes)
- String sponges
- Sponge forceps/clamp
- Rochester-Pean clamp
- Mayo clamp
- Bozeman forceps

Evaluation Directions: Place the appropriate number indicating the student's proficiency for each element using the following rating scale:

3—PROFICIENT. Can perform the task. Meets minimum entry level.

2—PARTIALLY PROFICIENT. Can perform most of the task. Needs assistance. Needs constant supervision.

1—LIMITED. Can do a limited amount of the task. Must be told what to do. Needs extremely close supervision.

0—UNSATISFACTORY. Cannot perform the task. Lacks knowledge, skills, and critical thinking skills while performing the task.

Skills	Grade	Self-Assessment	Instructor Initial
1. Student selects the appropriate clamp for creating a sponge stick and prepares it correctly.	0 1 2 3		
2. Selects the appropriate clamp for mounting sponge dissectors and prepares each size correctly.	0 1 2 3		
3. When mounting string (tonsil) sponge, correctly orients the string.	0 1 2 3		
Total			

SCORE

9	Proficient
6–8	Partially Proficient—Needs Remediation
Below 6	Unsatisfactory—Not Passing

Comments:

_____

_____

_____

_____

Student Signature: _____

Instructor Signature: _____

Management of Wound Dressings

Student's Name: _____ Date: _____

Task: Student will demonstrate the correct technique for preparing wound dressings. Student should demonstrate the technique for preparing each of the items listed. Student may prepare dressings on sterile draped Mayo stand covered with a clean towel.

Equipment and Supplies:

- Sterile gloves
- Telfa pad
- Gauze 4 × 4s
- Montgomery straps
- ABD pad
- Gauze fluffs
- Compression bandage
- Rolled gauze bandage
- Gauze packing
- Steri-Strips
- Op-site dressing
- Skin adhesive
- Dressing forceps
- Bandage scissors
- Sterile cloth towels
- Paper tape

Evaluation Directions: Place the appropriate number indicating the student's proficiency for each element using the following rating scale:

3—PROFICIENT. Can perform the task. Meets minimum entry level.

2—PARTIALLY PROFICIENT. Can perform most of the task. Needs assistance. Needs constant supervision.

1—LIMITED. Can do a limited amount of the task. Must be told what to do. Needs extremely close supervision.

0—UNSATISFACTORY. Cannot perform the task. Lacks knowledge, skills, and critical thinking skills while performing the task.

Skills	Grade	Self-Assessment	Instructor Initial
1. Student correctly prepares components for a simple abdominal dressing.	0 1 2 3		
2. Correctly prepares ABD pad and Montgomery straps.	0 1 2 3		
3. Correctly prepares gauze fluffs.	0 1 2 3		
4. Correctly prepares for dressing using Steri-Strips with skin adhesive.	0 1 2 3		
5. Correctly prepares rolled bandages: rolled compression dressing and Kling gauze.	0 1 2 3		
6. Receives gauze packing from circulator using aseptic technique. Correctly prepares packing and presents it to surgeon with forceps.	0 1 2 3		

Skills	Grade	Self-Assessment	Instructor Initial
7. Correctly prepares op-site dressing.	0 1 2 3		
8. Demonstrates correct procedure for applying a flat abdominal dressing, including application of tape.	0 1 2 3		
9. Student maintains a clean sterile field during preparation and application of dressings.	0 1 2 3		
Total			

SCORE

27   Proficient

18–26   Partially Proficient—Needs Remediation

Below 18   Unsatisfactory—Not Passing

Comments:

_____

_____

_____

_____

Student Signature: _____

Instructor Signature: _____

Connect Drainage Systems

Student's Name: _____ Date: _____

Task: Student will demonstrate the correct techniques for connecting drainage systems: Hemovac, Jackson-Pratt, underwater chest seal, stoma pouch.

Equipment and Supplies:
- Hemovac drainage system
- Jackson Pratt drain
- Single use underwater chest seal
- Chest tube
- Stoma pouch
- Straight Mayo Scissors
- Draped Mayo stand
- Gown and gloves

Evaluation Directions: Place the appropriate number indicating the student's proficiency for each element using the following rating scale:

3—PROFICIENT. Can perform the task. Meets minimum entry level.

2—PARTIALLY PROFICIENT. Can perform most of the task. Needs assistance. Needs constant supervision.

1—LIMITED. Can do a limited amount of the task. Must be told what to do. Needs extremely close supervision.

0—UNSATISFACTORY. Cannot perform the task. Lacks knowledge, skills, and critical thinking skills while performing the task.

Skills	Grade	Self-Assessment	Instructor Initial
1. Student correctly assembles Hemovac drain for insertion in patient. Demonstrates correct procedure for connecting tubes and activating the drain.	0 1 2 3		
2. Student correct assembles Jackson Pratt drain. Demonstrates correct procedure for connecting tubes and activating the drain.	0 1 2 3		
3. Student correctly assembles underwater chest seal equipment. Demonstrates correct procedure for filling chambers and connecting tubes.	0 1 2 3		
4. Student correctly assembles supplies needed to apply a stoma pouch. Correctly prepares the pouch for application over the stoma.	0 1 2 3		
Total			

SCORE

12	Proficient
8–11	Partially Proficient—Needs Remediation
Below 8	Unsatisfactory—Not Passing

Comments:

_____

_____

_____

_____

Student Signature: _____

Instructor Signature: _____

Process Flexible Endoscope

Student's Name: _____ Date: _____

Task: Student will demonstrate the correct technique for cleaning and high level disinfection of flexible endoscope.

Equipment and Supplies:

- Soaking basin
- Cleaning brushes dedicated to particular instrument
- Cleaning cloths
- Enzymatic cleaner
- Detergent
- Syringe
- PPE
- Pressurized air hose
- Distilled water
- Mechanical endoscope disinfection system

Evaluation Directions: Place the appropriate number indicating the student's proficiency for each element using the following rating scale:

3—PROFICIENT. Can perform the task. Meets minimum entry level.

2—PARTIALLY PROFICIENT. Can perform most of the task. Needs assistance. Needs constant supervision.

1—LIMITED. Can do a limited amount of the task. Must be told what to do. Needs extremely close supervision.

0—UNSATISFACTORY. Cannot perform the task. Lacks knowledge, skills, and critical thinking skills while performing the task.

Skills	Grade	Self-Assessment	Instructor Initial
1. Student gathers needed equipment and supplies for pre-cleaning according to manufacturer's instructions for use (IFU) at the point of use.	0 1 2 3		
2. Student performs precleaning correctly according to the manufacturer's IFU. Performs leak testing as required.	0 1 2 3		
3. Transports the endoscope correctly to the disinfection area; correctly maintains the endoscope and accessories in separate closed containers with appropriate biohazard label.	0 1 2 3		
4. Student dons PPE and correctly performs leak tests as required according to the manufacturer's IFU.	0 1 2 3		
5. Student proceeds to the cleaning process; correctly performs each step according to manufacturer's IFU; follows IFU for cleaning solution concentration and dilution factor, temperature, and water quality.	0 1 2 3		
6. Inspects the instrument correctly for debris or damage.	0 1 2 3		
7. Student proceeds to high level disinfection or sterilization using a mechanical processing unit or liquid sterilant.	0 1 2 3		

Skills	Grade	Self-Assessment	Instructor Initial
8. Student monitors the mechanical system to ensure that cycles are completed as required.	0 1 2 3		
9. Student stores the endoscope according to facility policy and manufacturer's IFU.	0 1 2 3		
10. Correctly documents the reprocessing procedure.	0 1 2 3		
Total			

SCORE

30	Proficient
20–29	Partially Proficient—Needs Remediation
Below 20	Unsatisfactory—Not Passing

Comments:

_____

_____

_____

_____

Student Signature: _____

Instructor Signature: _____

Fluid Pump for Continuous Irrigation

Student's Name: _____ Date: _____

Task: Student should show proficiency in setting up pump for continuous irrigation system for arthroscopy or cystoscopy; attaching fluid bags; thread tubing through pump; start and stop the pump.

If a gravity system is used, student should demonstrate how to set up fluid bags and tubing.

Evaluation Directions: Place the appropriate number indicating the student's proficiency for each element using the following rating scale:

3—PROFICIENT. Can perform the task. Meets minimum entry level.

2—PARTIALLY PROFICIENT. Can perform most of the task. Needs assistance. Needs constant supervision.

1—LIMITED. Can do a limited amount of the task. Must be told what to do. Needs extremely close supervision.

0—UNSATISFACTORY. Cannot perform the task. Lacks knowledge, skills and critical thinking while skills performing the task.

Skills	Grade	Self-Assessment	Instructor Initial
1. Attach fluid bags to tubing	0 1 2 3		
2. Thread tubing into pump	0 1 2 3		
3. Bleed air from tubing	0 1 2 3		
4. Start and stop the pump; adjust rate	0 1 2 3		
5. Gravity system: attach bags to tubing and bleed air	0 1 2 3		
6. Attach tubing to instrument correctly	0 1 2 3		
7. Maintains strict aseptic technique throughout the procedures	0 1 2 3		

SCORE

21	Proficient
14–20	Partially Proficient—Needs Remediation
Less than 14	Limited/Unsatisfactory—Not Passing

Comments:

_____

_____

_____

_____

Student Signature: _____

Instructor Signature: _____

Flexible Endoscope threading instruments

Student's Name: _____ Date: _____

Task: Student should demonstrate how to guide instruments into the correct channels during flexible endoscopy. Student should demonstrate how to set up suction and irrigation and demonstrate their use with the endoscope.

Evaluation Directions: Place the appropriate number indicating the student's proficiency for each element using the following rating scale:

3—PROFICIENT. Can perform the task. Meets minimum entry level.

2—PARTIALLY PROFICIENT. Can perform most of the task. Needs assistance. Needs constant supervision.

1—LIMITED. Can do a limited amount of the task. Must be told what to do. Needs extremely close supervision.

0—UNSATISFACTORY. Cannot perform the task. Lacks knowledge, skills and critical thinking while skills performing the task.

Skills	Grade	Self-Assessment	Instructor Initial
1. Set up suction and irrigation for endoscope	0 1 2 3		
2. Demonstrate basic instruments required for suction, irrigation, and biopsy.	0 1 2 3		
3. Demonstrate how to pass flexible instruments into the correct endoscope channels while maintaining sterility.	0 1 2 3		
4. Demonstrate how to withdraw flexible instruments while maintaining their sterility.	0 1 2 3		
5. Demonstrate how to transfer a specimen to its container (brush biopsy and biopsy forceps)	0 1 2 3		

SCORE

15	Proficient
10–14	Partially Proficient—Needs Remediation
Less than 10	Limited/Unsatisfactory—Not Passing

Comments:

_____

_____

_____

_____

Student Signature: _____

Instructor Signature: _____

Imaging System for Minimally Invasive Procedures

Student's Name: _____ Date: _____

Task: Student to demonstrate proficiency in setting up a digital imaging system using all components. Student should point out safety features and care of the imaging system. The list below includes components of the imaging system to be demonstrated. The student should be able to identify each component by name *and correctly connect each.*

Evaluation Directions: Place the appropriate number indicating the student's proficiency for each element using the following rating scale:

3—PROFICIENT. Can perform the task. Meets minimum entry level.

2—PARTIALLY PROFICIENT. Can perform most of the task. Needs assistance. Needs constant supervision.

1—LIMITED. Can do a limited amount of the task. Must be told what to do. Needs extremely close supervision.

0—UNSATISFACTORY. Cannot perform the task. Lacks knowledge, skills and critical thinking while skills performing the task.

Skills	Grade	Self-Assessment	Instructor Initial
1. Surgical telescope or endoscope	0 1 2 3		
2. Camera head	0 1 2 3		
3. Camera control unit (CCU)	0 1 2 3		
4. Light source and standby mode	0 1 2 3		
5. Light cable(s)	0 1 2 3		
6. Video cables	0 1 2 3		
7. Monitor	0 1 2 3		
8. Image management system (documentation system)	0 1 2 3		
9. Able to demonstrate procedure for white balancing	0 1 2 3		

SCORE

27	Proficient
18–26	Partially Proficient—Needs Remediation
Less than 18	Limited/Unsatisfactory—Not Passing

Comments:

_____

_____

_____

_____

Student Signature: _____

Instructor Signature: _____

Brown Dermatome

Student's Name: _____ Date: _____

Task: Prepare Brown dermatome including blade assembly; set level to 0.

Evaluation Directions: Place the appropriate number indicating the student's proficiency for each element using the following rating scale:

3—PROFICIENT. Can perform the task. Meets minimum entry level.

2—PARTIALLY PROFICIENT. Can perform most of the task. Needs assistance. Needs constant supervision.

1—LIMITED. Can do a limited amount of the task. Must be told what to do. Needs extremely close supervision.

0—UNSATISFACTORY. Cannot perform the task. Lacks knowledge, skills and critical thinking while skills performing the task.

Skills	Grade	Self-Assessment	Instructor Initial
1. Prepare Brown dermatome including blade assembly; set level to 0.	0 1 2 3		

SCORE

3	Proficient
2	Partially Proficient—Needs Remediation
Less than 2	Limited/Unsatisfactory—Not Passing

Comments:

_____

_____

_____

_____

Student Signature: _____

Instructor Signature: _____

Fit drill chuck or K-wire to keyed and keyless drill chuck

Student's Name: _____ Date: _____

Task: Student should demonstrate proficiency in attaching and detaching accessories to a keyed and keyless drill chuck.

Evaluation Directions: Place the appropriate number indicating the student's proficiency for each element using the following rating scale:

3—PROFICIENT. Can perform the task. Meets minimum entry level.

2—PARTIALLY PROFICIENT. Can perform most of the task. Needs assistance. Needs constant supervision.

1—LIMITED. Can do a limited amount of the task. Must be told what to do. Needs extremely close supervision.

0—UNSATISFACTORY. Cannot perform the task. Lacks knowledge, skills and critical thinking while skills performing the task.

Skills	Grade	Self-Assessment	Instructor Initial
1. Attach and detach drill accessories in a keyed drill chuck.	0 1 2 3		
2. Attach and detach drill accessories in a keyless drill chuck.	0 1 2 3		
3. Demonstrate use of safety lock on pneumatic and other powered drills.	0 1 2 3		
4. Demonstrate procedure for bleeding (draining) a pneumatic drill.	0 1 2 3		

SCORE

12	Proficient
8–11	Partially Proficient—Needs Remediation
Less than 8	Limited/Unsatisfactory—Not Passing

Comments:

_____

_____

_____

_____

Student Signature: _____

Instructor Signature: _____

Power Saw

Student's Name: _____ Date: _____

Task: Student should show proficiency in assembling components of a power saw including oscillating, reciprocal, and saggital blades.

Evaluation Directions: Place the appropriate number indicating the student's proficiency for each element using the following rating scale:

3—PROFICIENT. Can perform the task. Meets minimum entry level.

2—PARTIALLY PROFICIENT. Can perform most of the task. Needs assistance. Needs constant supervision.

1—LIMITED. Can do a limited amount of the task. Must be told what to do. Needs extremely close supervision.

0—UNSATISFACTORY. Cannot perform the task. Lacks knowledge, skills and critical thinking while skills performing the task.

Skills	Grade	Self-Assessment	Instructor Initial
1. Shows proficiency in attaching blades to power saw	0 1 2 3		

SCORE

3	Proficient
2	Partially Proficient—Needs Remediation
Less than 2	Limited/Unsatisfactory—Not Passing

Comments:

_____

_____

_____

_____

Student Signature: _____

Instructor Signature: _____